She Wrote it Down

HOW A SECRET-KEEPER BECAME A STORYTELLER

Laura Parrott Perry

ISBN: 0692048103
ISBN 13: 9780692048108

This book is for those who've made the decision to turn toward the sun,
and for those who are still in the darkness.

I see you.

Table of Contents

Foreword

by Matt Bays

I'VE DRAWN PICTURES of Snoopy since I was in third grade. If we received a one hundred percent on a spelling test, our teacher, Miss Schroeder, would draw a Snoopy in the upper, right-hand corner of our worksheet. I was a pretty good speller, so whenever I saw a Snoopy on my paper, I would trace Miss Schroeder's rendition and then work to perfect my own at home.

Before long, my mom caught on and Snoopy became the gift of choice for birthdays and Christmas. My favorite was a stuffed Snoopy doll with a radio in his belly. I took him to bed each night and listened to the music of the late 70's, early 80's until I fell asleep.

When you're a kid, it is mostly about the *sound* of the song—about how we feel when we hear it. In those days, most of us never paid attention to the lyrics, so they never found their way inside us.

In 1984, I joined the junior high wrestling team. I was thirteen years old. I was a good little wrestler, which I've always attributed to growing up in a house where I had to fight. With so much tension in my family of origin, to release the valve on the pressure-cooker, we fought. And I was good at it. I was a good little fighter.

Along my journey, I've found other good little fighters. On January 20th, 2015, I came across the blog, "In Others' Words" by Laura Parrott Perry. I remember the feeling as I read; the sacred space of authenticity that isn't trying to be well-mannered. The heartbreak of a demanding story, told with a measure of levity.

I read Laura's article twice, shared it on my feed, and left a comment on her post.

And she responded.

After that, I read everything she wrote. I was drawn in by her unique writing style that acknowledged the very real darkness of this world (not minimizing a single thing) but never once came off as terminal. There was always hope. Always lightness and joy. But also, always a sincere reverence for the places we don't like to talk about. Simply put, Laura made me feel like I could tell the truth and not die.

Since then, we've become friends. Like, actual friends. And I couldn't be more grateful. Because this little fighter needed a companion on the journey, and Laura has been that for me. Her ability to stand in her truth has helped me stand further into mine. Because there was more to my story, so much that still hadn't been told.

You see, after my wrestling practices, we would hit the showers; something that was equally exciting and shameful for me. With all its naked boys, the locker room was the place in the world that I most wanted to be. And yet, it was also a place of deep and impenetrable shame.

It seemed as if the other boys had been born in the locker room—as if the locker room was the womb where they'd been knit together. They had conversations about wrestling while soaping under their arms in the gang shower. They laughed at the dirty jokes teenage boys make while snapping towels at each other. It was a scene from High School Musical that had been choreographed in my absence. The whole wrestling team walked through their steps effortlessly, while I was an understudy who hadn't been prepped for the performance. I was a foreigner among the indigenous male adolescents of that locker room. And if I didn't belong there, I didn't belong anywhere.

I had already learned what it was to keep a secret. But at Northwood Junior High School, I learned that *who I was*, was the real secret to be kept.

In *She Wrote It Down*, Laura tells us, *We build our lives out of story and when we decide those stories are unspeakable, we build prisons out of our secrets.*

Fast-forward three and a half decades, and I'm living proof that Laura is (so painfully) right.

At this very moment, I'm sitting in an empty house. It's my new beginning that is filled with fear and what-ifs and what-the-hell-just-happeneds. I am alone and afraid. I am starting over. A new chapter or new story; I'm not sure which.

The last eleven months have altered my life in ways I never saw coming. I'm divorced from a woman I have loved for over two decades. I've come out as a gay man. My publisher put my book out of print because of my sexuality. My family has fallen apart and is desperately trying to rebuild.

Pain, tears, lies, regret.

Secrets.

When Laura asked me to write this foreword, I was certain it wasn't a good idea. I was convinced it had the potential of being the worst foreword to a book, ever; because I've got nothing to say about living an honest life, or holding it together.

But then I began reading *She Wrote It Down*, and Laura told me I didn't have to know something fool proof about life. She told me I was allowed to keep secrets, so long as those secrets found a writing table within me where they could begin the arduous process of turning themselves into stories. For the good of myself…and eventually, for the good of humankind.

I am impossibly grateful for this book. I laughed so hard while reading, only to have my eyes fill with tears fifteen seconds later.

And mystically, Laura was there the whole time. Because *She Wrote It Down* isn't a book, really, so much as a companion. She was with me in my living room, in the laundromat, sitting in a cold garage because I needed to finish this one last chapter.

In it, she never tells us 'how to' …because haven't we had enough of that already? Instead, she tells us…

I see you.

In eighth grade, I only wish someone had seen me. Because I was standing on very timid legs at the precipice of manhood, but I didn't know how to jump. And I needed help.

I had wrestled myself all the way to a city championship match. I was a strong boy who knew how to fight. But at night, I was still sleeping with stuffed animals.

You can't change the past, people say. Yes, I know. I've heard it all my life. But oh, my friend…can't we?

My favorite song in those days was *We Belong,* by Pat Benatar. Maybe it was her effortless vocals. Maybe it was the children's choir at the end of the song.

Or maybe it was the lyrics.

I'm standing at the door of my old bedroom on Crestview Drive. I'm looking across the room at the abused boy laying in his bed, wondering who the hell he is. Gay? Straight? A fraud of a boy? I tip toe toward him until I'm standing over his 92lb frame. For a moment, I watch him sleep, hugging the neck of a toy he has long outgrown.

I hear the song rising from his belly. This time, I let the lyrics wash over me. They are finding their way inside.

I kneel down next to him. I want to sing his favorite song to him. Because I know if I do, that one day he will find the strength to tell his secrets, to move forward…

to write it down.

I brush his hair back and smile. He is beautiful. Worth it. He is not alone. His chest floats up and down as I steal a breath of air from the past and whisper these perfect words into his ear.

Many times I tried to tell you
Many times I cried alone
Always I'm surprised how well I cut your feelings to the bone
Don't want to leave you really
I've invested too much time to give you up that easy
To the doubts that complicate your mind

We belong to the light, we belong to the thunder
We belong to the sound of the words we've both fallen under
Whatever we deny or embrace, for worse or for better
We belong, we belong
We belong together

My friends, so many of us are longing for things to be made right. Longing to be whole. And maybe in this collective longing, this is how we BE-long. For we are no longer secret keepers, hiding away all by ourselves. Not at all. We are storytellers. And we are writing it down.

Thank you, Laura. You wrote it down. And we believe you…that we are not alone.

None of us. Because we belong.

Together.

Introduction

"What would happen if one woman told the truth
about her life?
The world would split open."

Muriel Rukeyser

PUBLIC SPEAKING USED to terrify me. In order to stand in front of people and talk I needed to have planned out and memorized exactly what I was going to say. My heart would pound and my knees would buckle. I'd inhale unsteadily and race through what I needed to say. I'd find myself short of breath by the end.

I had to glaze my eyes over or look at some fixed point so I wasn't looking at people's faces. It was pure performance and I would intentionally disconnect from the audience in order to maintain my composure. It's tricky to be on stage and not be seen, but I'm pretty sure I pulled it off.

These days, I frequently find myself speaking in front of crowds. Sometimes it's on a large stage and sometimes it's in a tent at a festival. Sometimes it's in a circle of busted up folding chairs in a church basement.

My opening might vary a bit, depending on why I've been invited, but it is nearly always some version of the following:

Hi! My name is Laura Parrott Perry and I am a survivor of child sexual abuse. I'm also a recovering alcoholic, anorexic, and bulimic. I've basically got all your 'icks' covered.

I'm great at parties. Honest.

This guacamole's fabulous! Wanna talk trauma history?

I don't lead with those facts for the shock value or because they are the most important things about me or the most interesting. They're not. They are also no longer the way I define myself. I'm a woman, a mother, a writer, an activist, and an artist.

I lead with those particular facts for two reasons: First, I know the statistics for all those identifiers. When I scan the room, I immediately do the math. If I have a group of a hundred people, I know the numbers tell me that there are likely upwards of twenty survivors of sexual abuse, ten or more people who struggle with substance abuse, and at least three with disordered eating. Within that particular set of statistics there is an awful lot of overlap - I am living proof.

We all feel alone in those things. It's in the very nature of those struggles to believe it's just you, so it is always my intention to have as little time as possible pass between when I start talking and other people stop feeling alone in their pain.

Second, those stories were my shame stories and I have learned at long last and at great cost that shame needs to be dragged into the light. Shame requires the darkness of secrecy the way flowers require sunlight. It feeds on it.

Every time I give voice to those stories their grip on me lessens. Every time I tell what happened shamelessly, I take back control of my own narrative.

I have learned that for me, shame is like kryptonite. It was utterly destructive, a boot on my neck for most of my life. It is powerful and treacherous, and it is a luxury I cannot afford.

Our stories hold immeasurable power - all of them, whether they're narratives of triumph or shame. Our shame stories, though, wield power differently in the darkness and the light. When we are vulnerable and share those stories, we create a safe space for others to do the same. Those stories foment connection and community. Our shared stories of pain help us to identify with one another and to feel less alone in the world. Our untold shame stories have prodigious power, too.

Let's imagine a museum for a minute. What would we think of an exhibit kept cordoned off and hidden away? What would we make of something set behind velvet ropes and under special dim lighting, that few, if any, people were allowed to go back and witness? And what if those who were granted access had to pass all kinds of litmus tests, wear special gloves, and promise never speak of what they saw? What would we think of that exhibit compared to, say, one open to the general public?

I imagine we'd assume it was a pretty valuable exhibit, right? And if that was the ONLY artifact treated that way? The only relic locked away from prying eyes, the only piece afforded that much secrecy and security? One would naturally assume it to be the most valuable treasure of the whole lot.

Now imagine that your life is the museum and your stories are the exhibits.

When we treat our shame stories that way, when we hide them away, we assign them greater value. We treat them as though they are precious. Our refusal to give voice to our shame stories renders them more valuable, more powerful than our stories of love, redemption, and triumph.

When my stories went underground, when I guarded them closely, I made them dark treasures. I was constantly vigilant against encroachment on my secrets - if anyone got too close or pried too much I would double the security. I'd pull away. I'd lie. I'd perform.

I thought if I made myself invaluable, if I was good enough, or did enough, or gave enough - proved myself an essential asset, somehow - it would offset the shadowy deficit column of my shame stories. It never worked though. I always came up short. The scales were never balanced.

When I think about that it reminds me of the show Shark Tank. You know, when some young entrepreneur comes in and asks for $500K for 2% of his brand new company that has earned all of $132 dollars, and the Sharks blanch and say, *Your valuation is insane. How did you come up with that? Your company is not worth that much.* My valuation of my shame stories was insane, but because they were secrets I'd never allowed anyone to check my math.

When you have something that valuable, something that requires so much protection, your entire life is in service to its care and concealment. When my stories were hidden away, they were in charge of my whole life. I am a firm believer if your story is going untold to anyone, anywhere, that's not privacy, that's secrecy. Privacy and secrecy are not the same things.

Not every story needs to be told to everyone, not every fact of your life needs to be dragged into public. There's a difference, though, between choosing not to tell a particular story in a particular forum, and believing your story is unspeakable. The difference between privacy and secrecy is shame.

If you have a story that is hidden away, that you are unwilling or unable to share in any way, with anyone, anywhere, then it is the most powerful chapter in the story of your life. And the thing about shame is this: it is singularly malignant. And, like all good cancers, it does not stay contained. It metastasizes. It spreads. It conquers.

Our stories are insistent - they demand to be told. If you do not tell your story it will find a way to tell itself. Believe it.

If I reflect on the chapters in my life when I have been in despair, when I've suffered and struggled the most, there was a common denominator: a shame story that was going untold. Shame begets secrecy begets harmful coping behavior begets more shame: a toxic, hopeless spiral.

I spent forty-four years keeping secrets of one kind or another. All shame stories. Decades of hiding and lying and hustling lead me to a place of profound brokenness. I heard Rob Bell define despair as the belief that tomorrow will be exactly like today. That resonated deeply with me. When I hit rock bottom that's exactly how I felt. *This can never change*, and also, *I cannot do this for one more day.*

Because I'd deemed my stories unspeakable, I felt stuck, paralyzed. Our untold stories are static. They're not open to challenge, they can't be re-framed, they cannot be re-written.

My shame stories were a prison with an open door. I sat inside my shame, believing it was a dark, impenetrable fortress when all I needed to do was stand up and walk into the sunlight.

CHAPTER 1

In Others' Words

*"Come with your messy past. Come with your
uncertain future.
Come with your story you think no one
wants to hear...
Come as you are. Just come as you are."*

Rachel Macy Stafford

IT WOULD BE easy to say that my life turned around when I got sober - and it did. Of course. But I'd begun to save my life a year earlier.

In July of 2014, I was having a phone conversation with a friend. I was telling her how the time when I was struggling with my anorexia the most was the point in my life when I got the most frequent positive feedback from other women about the way I looked, and her reply was, *OOH. That should be your first book.*

M'kay. That's aggressive, I thought.

First book? And also, *book*?

I've always written. Well, that's not completely true, I suppose. I've always been a writer, I haven't always written. I had a good, solid decade of not writing.

I wrote (terrible) poetry and song lyrics when I was young, I wrote short stories for my kids when they were little. I took creative writing in college and loved it. I even got the high praise from a bro in my class that I could, *really write, for a girl.* Hard to believe with an affirmation like that I didn't just chuck all my other plans and start writing the Great American Novel. Bless.

Writing has always been how I process things. I frequently don't know what I think or believe about something until I write about it.

In any case, at a certain point, I just stopped. I was entrenched in the daily practice of mothering and being a wife. My world got really small for a long time, and I sort of lost my sense of who I was outside of who I loved.

I started writing again around the time I got divorced, mostly long Facebook posts, either about what was going on in the world or, eventually, what was going on in my life. Just parts of the truth, though. Little corners of it. Glimmers. And I was desperately lonely.

I began to open up to friends I'd made on the internet. I found an on-line community of people who seemed to be talking about real things. It felt safer, somehow, to share there with strangers. I could offer up a little piece of myself, be a little vulnerable, and then not have to see the person in the aisle at Trader Joe's or at a PTA meeting.

I decided to start blogging as a creative outlet. I was feeling untethered. I'd moved from Seattle back to the east coast, left my job, my established life. I was on the other side of my divorce and all that wreckage, but in the wake of it I'd created even more due to my drinking. I felt stuck. I was hovering between lives. The roles I'd formerly excelled at were defunct or seemingly irreparably damaged and I had no idea what to do with myself.

I launched my blog, In Others' Words, in October of 2014. I decided that since I had no idea what I wanted to write about or what my niche would be (other than NOT MOMMY BLOGGER) I would use the conceit of having an inspiration quote for each post. The unifying theme would be other writers' words, which would leave me open to write about anything I wanted.

Therefore, my first post was about my dog and the Dalai Lama. I mean... obviously.

Over the course of that first month, I wrote about friendship and art and my divorce, tattoos, eating disorders, and justice. I found the posts that resonated with my readers (all 43 of them) were the ones that brushed up against my shame stories. I wasn't telling WHOLE truths, but I was edging around them.

On the day I published my first post, I received a Facebook message from Deb, a woman I knew from Seattle. She said there was a conference coming up at the end of the month that I might be interested in. When she mentioned the name of it, my interest was immediately piqued.

Storyline.

I'd just told my first story publicly. It seemed serendipitous. I immediately felt as though this was something I was supposed to attend. I was in a season of saying yes to things (there was a fair amount of wine involved in my decision-making process back then) so I registered without giving it much thought. Then she told me one of my favorite writers was scheduled to speak. I thought, *Oh, well that's why I am supposed to go.*

When I saw it was in Chicago, a city I love and felt as though I lost in my divorce, I thought, *That's why I am supposed to go! I'm supposed to reclaim Chicago!* I still had no earthly idea what the conference really was - but I didn't so much care. I honestly didn't even really read the write-up. I felt that little buzz of certainty. Or maybe it was pinot. It's hard to say.

I kept having those moments of knowing throughout the conference. When I heard the brilliant spoken word artist Propaganda, the room was electrified and I wept at the beauty of his words. It seemed plausible he was why I was there. I walked over to a friend and we both said, *I can't even talk about it.*

When I heard Bob Goff speak I could NOT stop smiling. Is it possible for someone to have a carbonated soul? The room felt bubbly with joy the longer he spoke. I thought, *Clearly, I am here because I needed a little Bob Goff in my life.*

I heard Shauna Niequist implore us with words of wisdom that are hanging above my desk as I write this, and have served as a creative call to arms for me ever since – *Do YOUR THING, with GREAT LOVE, RIGHT NOW.*

Those were all great, life-altering experiences - but they were not why I was in Chicago that chilly October. I was in Chicago for two reasons.

I was at Storyline to hear Donald Miller say the words, *What will the world miss if you don't tell your story?*

I know.

It's a great line.

The thing is, it didn't feel like just a line. It didn't seem like a slogan or a catchphrase. It didn't seem rhetorical. It felt like a question being asked of me. It seemed like a question that required an answer.

I straightened up in my chair the first time he said it. I was afraid to look to my right or my left. I didn't want to make eye contact with anyone. I felt shaken. I felt exposed. I felt awake.

There were no bad speakers at Storyline. I took something away from each and every session. But the thing that kept creeping into my head during other talks, while I was eating, and while I was lying in bed, the thing I could not shake was, *What will the world miss if you don't tell your story?* The funny thing is, for a long time my answer would have been,

Nothing. Not one thing.

On the second night of the conference, my newfound friends and I were having a late dinner at the hotel bar. We were talking about the day and looking at the workbook we'd been given. The next day's lunchtime reflection questions were, *What is the most painful experience of your life?* and *While tragedy is something to be grieved, it can be redeemed. How is your tragedy also a blessing to you or others?*

Just a few lighthearted prompts over sandwiches and chips.

I decided to answer the first question - I did not have the answer to the second, yet.

I sat in that bar with three women I barely knew and I told them my story.

It was the first time I ever said out loud, *I am a survivor of sexual abuse.* That's the second reason I was at Storyline. I was there to sit with those three amazing women and tell that particular truth. Shamelessly.

I am a survivor.

For the first time ever, I didn't cry telling my story. For the first time ever, telling my story didn't put me back in my story. I wasn't triggered, I wasn't judging my younger self. I could look back on that little girl and feel empathy and compassion - I could feel outraged on her behalf - but I wasn't her anymore.

The next morning, I woke up with a vulnerability hangover. Also, an actual hangover. I had a little uneasiness about having shared my story, but it felt right. It felt like a beginning. I had the feeling it was time to write it down.

I didn't do it right away. There were some people in my life I needed to tell personally first. I needed to do some hard thinking and a lot of praying. I knew I needed to be quiet with it before I laid myself bare like that. Sometimes that comes at a cost. I didn't know what my family's reaction would be. Once you put something out into the world you don't have any control over what happens to it and you need to be prepared for whatever reaction it elicits. I didn't fully appreciate how true that was, yet. I did, however, trust I would know when the time was right.

It wouldn't leave me alone, though. That question followed me around, day after day, nipping at my heels.

What will the world miss if you don't tell your story?

I might've stayed stuck in that indefinitely had the Universe not conspired to get me moving. On Thanksgiving morning, not three weeks after Storyline, I woke up to a friend request on Facebook from my cousin Mary.

I'd thought of Mary so many times over the years - my sisters and I were so close with her when we were little, but it had been three and a half decades since we'd had any contact. I disclosed my abuse and we basically never saw that side of our family again. I felt a visceral flash of fear. I didn't know what she wanted or what she remembered or what she thought of me. And, why now? I was nervous, but I decided to trust my gut and I accepted her request.

Then, I did what any sane person would do; I low-grade stalked her on social media. I snooped around her Facebook profile. She was gorgeous. So was her husband. So were their kids. So was their dog. She seemed pretty fancy.

It wasn't long before she messaged me. We chatted back and forth a bit, and in short order we found ourselves on the phone. Our first conversation lasted three and a half hours. The awkwardness dissipated immediately. We both cried. Soon, it was as though no time had passed. There were so many parallels in our lives, lots of *me too* moments. About an hour and a half in, Mary expressed sorrow and confusion as to why we were separated, why we were torn from each other. She said, *I know your parents got divorced, but people get divorced - you don't just lose your whole family! You don't just never see each other again!*

The hot fear bubbled up in me. Things were going so well. I wasn't sure I was ready to derail everything by telling her the real reason. I didn't know what she knew or remembered, so I hedged. I said,

Well, I think there were lots of reasons...

It was a long couple of seconds.

Then Mary said, *Let's talk about the elephant in the room.* So we did. She disclosed to me that our grandfather had abused her, too. I knew this on some level, but nevertheless, it was a painful homecoming. *Me too.* Two more hours of connecting dots, filling in missing pieces, realizing how similarly the abuse had played out in our lives even given the differences of how our story was handled, followed.

I got off the phone somehow simultaneously depleted and filled up.

It would be another month and a half before I was ready to write publicly about my abuse, but one day, in early January, I posted an essay called, *The Fault in my Scars.*

In the course of a few short months, I went from being a life-long secret-keeper to a fledgling storyteller. That sent into motion a chain of events that would radically alter the trajectory of my life; it would heal me, make clear my purpose, and it would send me hurtling toward rock bottom and sobriety.

CHAPTER 2

Hush

"No one keeps a secret so well as a child."

Victor Hugo

WHEN MY KIDS were tiny I would play a game with them where I would whisper something silly in their ear and then admonish them, *Now, DON'T TELL ANYONE!!!* Of course, they would begin to giggle and immediately rat me out to whoever else was in the room:

Daddy, Mommy said you're SILLY!

Cue the hysterical giggling that inevitably follows such sanctioned disobedience.

It was along the same lines of coaxing a truculent child to lighten up, *Don't you DARE SMILE,* knowing full well the end result will likely be a grudging and, eventually, delighted grin, just to spite you. The whole point of the game was a secret not kept.

I wonder if in some small part that's because I did not want my kids to get comfortable with secrecy.

I became a secret keeper at the age of eight. What does eight years old look like? Well, it looks like scraped knees and Barbie dolls. It looks like a flowered basket on the front of your bike and four-square at recess. It looks like believing in the Tooth Fairy and that the moon follows your car home at night.

And knowing that monsters are real.

Before that age I'd kept some secrets, but that's the year I learned how high a price you can pay for speaking the truth. When I finally got to the point where my fear of not telling was greater than my fear of telling, I confided in my mother that I was being sexually abused by my paternal grandfather.

While that disclosure meant that I was physically safe from that point on, I learned that simply saying what happened can cleave your world in two. I learned that asking for help carried with it an enormous risk.

So I stopped. I stopped telling the truth. I stopped asking for help. I learned that in most cases, *How are you?* was a rhetorical question, and the preferred answer was, *FINE!* I learned which version of me was the most pleasing and I wore her like a costume. I learned to hide the anger that practically radiated off me under humor and smiles and deference.

When I got to college that became more challenging. Alcohol became a regular part of my life - and I'll be honest, that felt like a blessing from God. I had my first drink at eleven and drank periodically in high school, but it didn't become a regular thing until I left home.

You know when someone is in dire pain in the hospital and they're put on a morphine drip with the button they can click when they need relief? That's what having easy access to alcohol felt like. Pain. Drink. Relief. Anger. Drink. Relief. Fear. Drink. Relief.

The problem was this - while one or two drinks calmed the anger, too many unleashed it - and I very seldom was able to stay in the one drink realm. Not by choice, anyway.

Pretty early on in my college experience, I got labeled a "b*tch." (Please note that I have zero problems swearing, but Brené Brown ruined that word for me forever, and I can't even fully type it now.) I remember seeing that movie About Last Night and while I knew on some level I was supposed to be rooting for Demi Moore's character, I was kind of obsessed with her perennially angry, unpleasant best friend played by so beautifully by Elizabeth Perkins.

I was quick to take offense and could nurture a resentment like nobody's business. I would assign intentions to people, never flattering, and then view everything they did through that lens. I was a great prosecutor for other people's offenses and a great defense attorney for my own.

I was a hard person to love in those years.

As my college years went on, my drinking got more problematic. My friends all drank a lot, and I don't know that my consumption ever stood out in terms of quantity - but the way I drank was always different. And I always seemed to have consequences that other people didn't have. I regularly found myself in dangerous situations, I found myself in conflict with people I cared about. I was headed for ruin.

I got pregnant my senior year and some tiny remnant of survival instinct took hold. If it had simply been a case of

self-preservation I don't know that I could have course-correct-
ed. I wanted to be a good mother more than anything else in
the world, though. I wanted my little family to make it, so I
stopped. Part of me felt guilty having a baby because I knew I
was a disaster. It felt selfish. But I loved him before he got here
and he saved my life in a hundred million ways. My son became
my sun.

And so, my drinking largely went into remission. I certainly
can't say I didn't drink during the next eighteen years, but for
a long time, I seldom did. When I did, though, it tended to go
sideways.

Let me be crystal clear about this point- I do not think the
circumstances of my life - my trauma, my divorce - made me an
alcoholic. I was more susceptible to picking up that first drink,
though. I was more inclined to look for escape. I have always
been an alcoholic, even when I wasn't drinking. I drank in response to those things *because* I am an alcoholic.

Until I got sober, I had never not lied about my drinking.
I always downplayed how much I'd had. If I had way too much
and blacked out, I would try and fake my way through, hoping
to piece things together enough to hide the fact I'd lost control. Again. I'd come up with reasons why I'd gone too far: I
was tired, hadn't eaten, and even (bless my heart) that I didn't
drink often enough to have built up a tolerance. I would power
through crushing hangovers and refuse to acknowledge them
even back in college when my friends practically luxuriated
in theirs, complaining epically about their misery like it was a
badge of honor.

What that tells me is that from a very young age I'd attached shame to my drinking. My unhealthy relationship with alcohol became another secret for me to keep. Another untold story. Another mask. The secret I used to manage my secrets.

CHAPTER 3

Sofas and Backseats

*"I had learned early to assume something dark and
lethal hidden at the heart of anything I loved. When
I couldn't find it, I responded, bewildered and wary in
the only way I knew how: by planting it there myself."*

Tana French

I'M SITTING IN the backseat of my mother's car heading home
from Cape Cod one summer night. I don't have the vocabulary
to fully convey what is happening to me. I don't understand it,
really. It's just that the thought of what might happen has become more frightening than the thought of the repercussions
of telling. Telling has simply become the lesser of two horrors.

My mother is understandably devastated and outraged. I
should feel better, having told, but I don't. I know I haven't told
everything. There are things I don't have words for yet. But if
this is the reaction to the partial truth, I understand the whole
truth is too dangerous to speak out loud. Some parts must be
tucked away. There are parts of my story that will remain untold
for another decade. Secrets are born.

I'm sitting in a family counseling session across from my father. I can feel the waves of rage emanating from him. It's as though I can see them, these cold, shimmery reverberations of fury. Not rage on my behalf, not rage at the harm done to his daughter. His rage is at me. He is enraged because he thinks I am lying or have been put up to it. I am holding my breath.

He doesn't believe me and I know it. If I could take it all back in this moment, I would. I remember reading the myth of Pandora's Box in school and flashing back to that moment. That's what it feels like. Like I've made this enormous error in judgment, like I've poisoned the air, our family, by opening my mouth and letting the truth escape.

⋅⊷▣◕ ◔▣⊶⋅

My lasting trauma began in that car and on that couch. Not on the walk with the dog, when my abuse began. Not in the pool cabana, or under the stairs where it continued. Not on the utility room floor, where it concluded in violence.

Don't get me wrong, all of those situations were traumatic - but until those two moments in the wake of telling my truth, my grandfather was a bad man, certainly, but I didn't necessarily believe the story he was telling me about myself or the world.

My abuser told me if I said anything there would be serious consequences, and to my child's mind that threat was borne out. By the way they reacted to my disclosure, the people in my life unwittingly made my grandfather a truth-teller. And because I was a child trying to make sense of something painful and complicated, I created a simple story out of a complex and confusing set of facts. I decided if he was right about that one thing, he was right about everything.

Human beings build homes out of story and they live in them. Kids, in particular, are naturally imaginative and creative. All human beings are, but children are less married to the concrete. Their thinking is more fluid, less developed - they don't know as much and have less life experience, so they aren't as encumbered by fact and perspective. So like primitive people, when there are gaps in their knowledge, or there is something they don't understand, they fill it in with story.

We make sense of our heartache and trauma the way ancient civilizations made sense of the world - with story. Primitive people did not understand weather or natural phenomena, so what did they do? They used story to explain it. They created gods and goddesses, rituals and rules. Human beings have never been comfortable in the liminal space of not-knowing. We are seekers. We would rather be sure about something that is patently untrue than sit with the discomfort of uncertainty.

For people living in villages alongside volcanoes many centuries ago, an eruption for no reason was too terrifying a reality in which to live. Lacking the scientific understanding of tectonic disruptions, magma, and physics, civilizations living next door to temperamental mountains combined a few facts, a little myth, and more than a soupçon of misogyny and decided that every so often a young woman of unimpeachable moral standards must be tossed inside to appease whatever deity was in charge of eruptions.

Now, did the volcano remain dormant because they made their annual virgin sacrifice? Of course not. Did any of that matter to the unfortunate girl tossed into the lava? Of course not. She lived and died out of a story someone else created for her. A confabulation. A story that is untrue, but believed by the teller. In the end, though, that poor girl wasn't any less dead because her sacrifice was predicated on a lie.

My childhood abuse was traumatic, yes. But the real trauma, the lasting harm, came from what I told myself about it, other people's reactions to me telling my story, and the conclusions I drew about the dangers of telling my story. My world felt fractured and unsafe. Once you've destabilized the foundation of someone's life it becomes fertile ground for the seeds of shame.

That's how shame gets introduced, and it is always introduced. Shame always comes from outside. It's never indigenous, it needs to be planted. Once it takes hold it doesn't require much tending. In fact, the quickest way to encourage shame to take root is to leave it all alone in the dark. Then it does what invasive species always do; it takes over, bit by bit, until it crowds out all that is natural and good and healthy. Unchecked, shame conquers.

So all of those lies my grandfather told me about myself, whether overtly or by the way he treated me and used my body, became true for me. I unquestioningly accepted them. You see, we humans don't use facts to shore up our stories, we use story to shore up the facts of our lives. We use story to make sense of the incomprehensible. We use story to combat the dissonance of trauma.

In the car, and later, on that dreary couch, I came to see my abuser as a reliable source of information. It was in those moments he became the author of my story. I stopped telling it and he started.

I learned valuable lessons from the way my story was handled and those lessons would color how I saw the world. I learned that in my family it was more important for things to look okay than to be okay. Well, I've always been a quick study.

Even though I'd spoken the truth, it went back underground. That felt like the safer choice. And because I wasn't giving voice to my experience, because I wasn't getting help with untangling the narrative of the story my abuser told me about myself, it went unchallenged. It went unchallenged and I lived as though it was true - and so eventually, much of it was.

I was called a liar. Well, what do liars do? They lie. So I lied, and then I was a liar. Now, lying can look like more than one thing. Lying can be telling overt untruths, which I certainly did, but it also can mean leaving a truth untold.

I was taught that my value lay in my sexuality before I even knew what that was, so I led with my sexuality. I learned that my *no* was not enforceable, so I stopped saying it. I believed I wasn't worthy of respect, so I gravitated toward people who agreed with me about that. I'd prayed to God to stop my abuse, and then to make my dad believe me. I believed those prayers went unanswered. The story I told myself about that was that God had forsaken me, and I lived accordingly.

Those were the stories I lived in, the secrets that became my prison. Those were my unspoken, unchallenged stories, and they informed the way I lived. So, play that through to the end. What did that look like in the life of a young girl? A teenager? A woman? A mother? A wife?

Well, it looked like my first drink at eleven. A suicide attempt at twelve. It looked like anorexia and bulimia - starving myself in an attempt to disappear. It looked like reckless promiscuity - seemingly inviting trauma to come my way again, and so over and over, it did. It looked like perfectionism and hustle and busyness and exhaustion. It looked like a paralyzing fear of failure, which was, and sometimes still is, only exceeded by my fear of success.

ALL of those things were my story being told, it was just my abuser telling it,

Our stories are insistent. They will make themselves known, one way or another.

There are tipping points in our lives and the story I told myself about my abuse and its aftermath was one of mine. It did not matter that absolutely none of it was true. I accepted it all as fact and lived accordingly. Those lies became the Gospel according to which I lived my life. The Bad News.

And when you believe those things about yourself, your family, and God?

Well, that profoundly changes the way you move through the world.

When I refused to tell my story, it would find ways to tell itself.

Chapter 4

The Absence of Light

"Darkness has a hunger that's insatiable,
and lightness has a call that's hard to hear."

Indigo Girls

We move through the world surrounded by story. Human beings are continuously crafting and telling our stories. Even as I live my own and pour it out, I take in other people's stories nearly every day.

Just about every morning, I wake up to someone's story in my inbox.

The emails are usually sent late at night. Something about the darkness, perhaps. Isn't that when we reflexively, even desperately, seek the light?

They generally start out with something akin to an apology. *Sorry to bother you with this, I know you hear these things all the time*, or *I don't know why I'm even sending this...*

They are primarily stories of harm. That may sound depressing. I probably would have thought that one point in time. It doesn't feel that way to me now, though. Somehow, I have come to be identified as a safe place for other people to lay down some heavy things. I'm not always certain whether these people are seeking anything in particular, or if carrying the unrelenting weight of their secrets alone simply becomes too much. Perhaps they're simply looking to relieve themselves of the burden for a minute or two or maybe they're just looking to be seen by someone.

There's an outside chance it doesn't matter.

Either way, odds are if I have an email in my blog inbox first thing in the morning, it is likely someone coming to me with their story of trauma.

It hasn't always been that way. I wasn't always the sort of person people instinctively thought of as a safe haven for their confidences. It's funny, back then I had so many well-kept secrets of my own, you would think that would inspire faith in someone looking to tell a hidden truth. What is that about, I wonder? The more secretive I was about my own pain, the less safe a place I was for other people's. The more open I am about my own secrets, the more people entrust me to safeguard theirs.

I was carrying around so many closely guarded shame stories, each neatly folded up with all the weight of a black hole collapsing in on itself. Impossibly heavy, impossibly dark. The kind of dark that stays on the move. The kind of dark that spreads and isn't content to just be dark itself - it needs to snuff out light wherever it finds it. A voracious darkness.

CHAPTER 5

Once Upon a Time

"You're a storyteller. Dream up something wild and improbable," she pleaded. "Something beautiful and full of monsters."
"Beautiful and full of monsters?"

"All the best stories are."

Laini Taylor

THE ONLY EXACT words I remember him saying to me are these:

Let me feel your little body.

I think I was probably seven. Memory is such a tricky thing, especially in childhood. I know I was young, even though I don't remember feeling that way. Ever.

Grampa knew I loved animals - I was crazy about them, so when he asked me to come with him while he walked the dog, Calamity, I naturally said yes.

I know. The irony is not lost on me. I went for a walk with calamity.

She was a collie, a really beautiful dog. I loved her so much. I remember walking down the long driveway. It was a languid summer afternoon. It was hot and humid. It was the kind of afternoon that would have benefitted from a sudden, violent thunderstorm to break the heaviness. I remember the way the dog lifted her elegant, pointy snout to sniff the air. I remember the way her long fur looked in the dappled sunlight as she trotted down the hill. I remember being excited that I got to go alone with him. He asked me. Not my sisters. ME. That had never happened before.

I felt singled out. Special.

I'd never had a particularly close or warm relationship with him the way I did with my mom's dad, my Pepa. Pepa always had a twinkle in his eye when he looked at me. He called me his Blue-Eyed Banditty. He loved to look up things in the encyclopedia to answer our questions, help us to identify birds and plants, be silly with us, make corny jokes. He delighted in us.

That was never the case with my father's dad. He just wasn't that sort of grandparent.

That first time is so clear in my memory. The angle of the light, the black-eyed Susans standing still in the breezeless field. I remember the little pond with the bridge. And then I remember a hand up my shirt. Then, one down my shorts.

I remember laughing at first. I thought he was trying to tickle me. I was notoriously ticklish. Then a big hand pulled me hard back up against him, his back to the house. Anyone looking down probably wouldn't have even been able to see me, I was so little, such a tiny, skinny thing. And then he said those words.

It felt weird. It felt dumb and weird and awkward. I wasn't scared, exactly. More confused than anything, I suppose. After a couple of minutes he said we should go back and that I shouldn't say anything. So I didn't.

That's the first incident I remember, although looking back I know that's not where it began. I have memories of being held in his lap against my will, squirming mightily to get away while he laughed and adults urged me to, *Give Grampa a kiss*. I remember him "accidentally" walking in on me in the bathroom and in the cabana while I was changing, over and over and over again. A series of little boundary violations, all seemingly innocent mistakes, easily explained away. In hindsight, nothing you could really put your finger on without sounding like you were making a big deal out of a misunderstanding.

I remember being in the basement sitting room with my cousin Mary and her cautioning me not to sit on Grampa's lap because he would try to stick his tongue in my mouth. I laughed. She was trying to warn me and I *laughed*. We've talked about it, and Mary doesn't remember that conversation. I do. I think about that moment often. It was the seventies and no one talked to kids about sex, especially not that young. I didn't know what I didn't know. I had no framework to understand what that was or why anyone would do that. It seemed ridiculous.

Once my abuse began in earnest, I knew that Mary could only know to warn me about that if it was happening to her, too. We never talked about it, though. We were a well-trained family. Secret-keepers being raised by secret-keepers.

I don't know how long it went on, or how many incidents there were. I have flashes of other times, memories that are more ephemeral. I remember running up the stairs, panicking because he was trying to grab my feet. I still run up open staircases, today. I remember struggling in the cabana, the low, buzzing hum of the pool generator and the overwhelming smell of chlorine.

And I remember the last time.

He asked me if I wanted to help feed the cat. For the life of me, I don't know why I fell for it. I remember everything about that time because that time was different.

That time I said *no*.

Before I said no, my abuse had been frightening and a little uncomfortable, but not painful and not violent - at least, I hadn't perceived it that way.

My saying no changed the dynamic. It didn't seem as though he was used to hearing that.

I remember the linoleum floor of the utility room. It was cold and hard.

I remember the cat's food dish by my head. To this day I can't smell wet cat food without gagging and feeling light-headed.

I remember being held down, a big forearm on my throat.

I remember the pain and the pushing. I didn't understand what was happening. I didn't know what sex was, but I was terrified. People always say rape is a fate worse than death. I can tell you, it's not. As terrifying and painful and awful as it was, I remember just wanting to live. That's all I remember thinking; I just didn't want to die and it felt like I might.

I remember the weight of him. He was so heavy.

I remember the smell of him - sweat and stale cigarette smoke. I remember he always breathed with his mouth open, as though he was panting.

I remember it was hard for me to breathe, so I held my breath. A tiny act of rebellion. If I wasn't going to breathe, it would be my choice.

Mostly, I remember he didn't look at me.

He never looked at me. His eyes were like the eyes of a shark. Blank. Flat.

Staring off at something else. Not angry, but not present, either. Just coldly, single-mindedly determined.

I remember afterward he said something to the effect that if I said anything people would be upset and angry and they wouldn't believe me. And then he left.

Later that night he came up to me in the kitchen. He put his hand on the top of my head and gave it a squeeze. It probably looked like a gesture of affection. I guarantee it was not.

I recall not wanting to be away from my sisters the next day. When my sisters weren't around I hovered close to my Nana. I remember her sitting outside – I think she was doing a cross stitch or something. I remember wanting to be in the pool because it felt safe, but I was bleeding and I didn't want anyone to know. I kept looking down at the clear blue water making sure it didn't show. I remember not sleeping all night.

I remember just wanting to go home.

Those are the facts of my abuse. They were traumatic and painful, but they are not why I struggled for decades with shame and self-loathing. They are not why I starved myself. They are not why I drank. They are not why abusive and toxic relationships felt so comfortable to me. They are not why, for the better part of my life, I came from a place of not enough. Why I was in perpetual hustle mode.

Those struggles were born of the story I built around the facts of my abuse. The facts were just the scaffolding of the house my story built. I dwelled in that story, living out of lies I'd been told and sold about myself, and devoting constant time and energy to keeping my secrets hidden.

CHAPTER 6

Enough

*"Sometimes I need
only to stand
wherever I am
to be blessed."*

Mary Oliver

THE FIRST TIME I drank with peers I was thirteen years old. It was a winter night and I was sitting in the backseat of a Camaro at a local parking spot that overlooked the ocean, because of course I was. I was that girl. I was with a friend who was my age and two much older boys. The air was thick with Drakkar Noir. It was the 80's and that was the law.

The whole night was drenched in the kind of excitement that seldom comes about in the absence of bad decisions - the slightly manic laughter of teenagers up to no good. I didn't live in a house of many rules but I'm pretty sure I was breaking all of them.

We were passing around an unholy concoction of chocolate milk and peppermint schnapps. It was nearly as good as it sounds.

Everyone in the car was having fun. Well, almost everyone. I was smiling and laughing because I knew what fun looked like and I have always been good at reading a room. Or a muscle car.

I wasn't having fun. I was keeping track. It was kind of stressful, actually.

Will the bottle come around again? Why is she drinking so much? Do we have a way to get more? I had hit that sweet spot. You know that place? I could feel that creeping warmth in my legs and I could feel my shoulders relax.

I just wanted to stay there. Right there. And for me to do that, there needed to be enough. I held my breath. I was very concerned with getting my share - getting what I needed to maintain that feeling.

I had not yet learned that enough was and would continue to be an illusion for me. That sweet spot was so freaking elusive. It was like trying to grab smoke or light and hold it in my hands. I would hit the mark - that moment when the fear and the anger and the shame seemed to melt away and I could breathe easy - and then I would overshoot or it would wear off. All I wanted to do was coast and breathe, but it seldom, if ever, worked out that way. It was too much or not enough, every damned time.

It's difficult for non-alcoholics to understand, I think. I was never trying to get drunk. Ever. I was trying to stay still. Particularly toward the end of my drinking days, I always had an active plan to not get drunk. I was trying to control something beyond my control. The truth for me is this: once alcohol is in my system, it does whatever the hell it wants with me.

I was keenly aware, even all those years ago sitting in that backseat, that I was having a different experience than the rest of my companions. That my relationship with alcohol, with drinking, was different than other people's.

I also instinctively knew to keep this a secret.

The funny thing about addiction is that you use your drug of choice to escape the present and then you chase it trying to stay present in your escape. The beautiful thing about sobriety is that all I need do to stay where I'm at is simply to stay where I am.

Sometimes that means staying still for uncertainty and discomfort, but it also means I get to stay still for joy and serenity. I stay where I'm at and wherever that is, whatever that looks like, I tell the truth about it.

There may have been an age when I was unfamiliar with worry, but I don't remember it. I grew up with scarcity. Actual scarcity. Lights and heat off during the winter in New England, scarcity. Non-functioning appliances, bare cupboard scarcity. I worried about it all the time. There never seemed to be enough.

I find that when I stay in the present in sobriety I do not worry about enough. If I time travel back to dark and cold days it leads to worry. If I'm projecting about how to put my kid through college, I worry.

If I stay right here, right now? Well, right here, right now, I have enough.

And the truth is, even back in the cold and the darkness I had enough. You know how I know that? I'm here.

It's another day at the beach, but I'm not thirteen anymore. More than thirty years have passed, but I am still the girl who likes to park at the beach. I'm by myself this time, though, and it's coffee in my cup. It's not sunny, but the sky is a bright grey. It's not warm, but it's okay. The water is choppy and opaque, and there's sort of an ominous energy to the water and sky. I love days like this, when something's brewing.

That's how I've been feeling, actually.

Something's brewing.

I've been aware of a lot of fear lately. I'm glad I recognize it now. I never really thought I was a fearful person. That's because my fear always wore disguises. My fear dressed up as anger, as control, as judgment.

Part of the beauty of doing the work of recovery is discovering what's at the root of your behavior patterns. I know today that I can sit still with fear. I can acknowledge it, name it, and then decide to be brave.

Today, I know that on the other side of fear is almost always something good. Maybe better. On the other side of whatever storm this is that's brewing will be sunshine and calmer waters.

I can sit with that. I can trust there will be enough.

Recently, during a hard week, I showed up at a meeting and we were locked out. I panicked. The feeling was exactly the same as it was back when I was drinking and needed more alcohol. *How will I get what I need to be okay?*

The fact of the matter is, had the door remained locked and the closest I got to that church basement was the unlit parking lot with my beautiful, mad community, that would have been enough.

I always, always have enough.

That's a gift of recovery. When things get hard, I know enough to head for church basements. Because I live near the ocean and God loves me, a few of those church basements take place on the beach.

I wake up to a stunningly beautiful autumn day. The sky is a deep blue and there are a few high, skittering clouds. It's not cold, but the air is crisp and full of energy, almost anticipation. When I get to the beach, the sand is covered in the tracks of the raucous gulls that come to scavenge for food.

By the time I leave, the sand has been further disturbed by a circle of beach chairs, blankets, and the footprints of my rowdy tribe, who show up mornings, rain or shine, just trying to survive.

We're all just looking for our daily bread.

CHAPTER 7

Disappearing Act

"I knew who I was this morning, but I've changed a
few times since then."

Lewis Carroll

SOMETIMES FACEBOOK MEMORIES feels like watching that first
scene in Jaws when the woman is in the water and you know
she's about to get jerked under. My posts from seven years ago
pop up and I think, *Oh. Bless her heart. Look how happy she is. She
has no freaking idea what's coming.* Then there are the pictures after
I'd been steamrolled.

You know the difference between those photos? Nothing. I
look almost exactly the same before and after. One such 'after'
post is a picture of me sitting in the gorgeous kitchen of my new
dream home. On the window behind me are snowflakes I'd cut
out with my kid and my niece and nephew; the last vestiges of
the Christmas decorations I was always loathe to take down.
My make-up is perfect. My hair is shiny and behaving, for once.
It's February of 2011, but February in the Pacific Northwest, so
the huge, glorious backyard the window looks out over is still
green. I have a big smile on my face.

I believe at that point I'd known for about a week that my life was imploding.

⤙▱ ▱⤚

In October of 2010, I'd just moved into my dream home. It was everything I'd ever wanted in a house. Actually, that's not true. It far exceeded anything I'd ever even dared dream to want in a house. We'd lived in the Seattle area for about seven years in our modest starter home. We'd lived pretty frugally, my husband had become quite successful, and we were ready to upgrade.

I'd been aware of the house for quite some time. We'd looked at it a few years prior. It was a disaster at that point. Every single surface needed to be redone. Fascinating paint colors, tragic carpet, awful countertops, but it was a beautiful house. So much potential. Great bones. It just needed to be fixed up on the surface. I was madly in love with it, but it was at the height of the housing market bubble, it was really expensive and made no sense to buy. I was crestfallen but my husband was right. It was a money pit.

Cut to a few years later. In the interim, a very nice family had purchased the house, completely renovated it, the housing market had crashed, we had that much more money saved, and the house was in reach.

We bought it and moved in. My picture-perfect, sprawling yellow Cape; my dream kitchen with its massive island and double oven; my fireplaces, my huge backyard. MY GAZEBO. I mean... it was a dream I'd not been audacious enough to have, come true. When my posts from that time come up on Facebook they are full of the words *lucky* and *grateful*. I was so, so lucky, and profoundly grateful for the life I'd somehow cobbled together. I couldn't believe the life I found myself living.

I felt like I'd finally hit my stride. I had two incredible kids, a stunning home, a perfect dog, a good marriage - not without its problems, certainly. I mean, I didn't really feel seen, and likely he didn't either, but we cared about each other and we'd built a life, you know?

I had a couple of close friends, plenty of people I called friends, I was a PTA fixture, I had volunteer work that filled me up. If you'd asked me, I'd have told you I was living an amazing life.

In December of that year, I turned forty. The doorbell rang one morning, and it was my sister from San Diego. My husband had flown her in as a surprise for my birthday. The next day, three dear friends from the east coast arrived. It was blessing, upon blessing, upon blessing.

There are photos from that weekend of me, surrounded by people I love, glasses raised, with a huge smile on my face.

I kept thinking, *I cannot believe this is my life.*

Then the bottom dropped out and for four years I disappeared. Well, I gave it my best effort, anyway.

Shortly after that birthday, I discovered my marriage was not what I'd believed it to be. The details don't matter anymore, really. That sort of realization causes a palpable shift to take place. I lost my center of gravity. Literally. I felt unsteady on my feet. I walked around in a daze, dispassionately observing myself from the outside. I lived in a beautiful house, in a beautiful neighborhood, with two beautiful children and a beautiful dog. And this thing, this ugly, cancerous truth had been introduced into our lives.

Everything was topsy-turvy. I was Alice in Wonderland, and I just wanted to get home - to exit the rabbit hole and go back to not knowing.

The night I found out, I skipped dinner, took a bottle of red out of the fancy wine refrigerator, and went upstairs to my room. The thought of eating was ridiculous. The thought of feeling, even more so. I was aiming for numb. I hit the mark.

I gave myself permission. I felt entitled to the anesthesia.

The next morning, I made breakfast for the kids. My husband tried to hug me on his way out the door and I stood frozen in my lovely kitchen. I sent the kids off to school and went about my day. I skipped breakfast. Lunch made no sense to me. I felt like I was trying to walk through Jell-o. Everything was so heavy. At dinner, I pushed food around my plate hoping that the kids would think I was eating. I felt empty and that felt appropriate. I was empty.

I kept forgetting to breathe. I wouldn't notice until I was gasping for breath.

And the hits kept coming. Little aftershocks of information trickled in, jarring me, causing more fissures in the foundation. Everything I learned seemed to challenge a truth I'd held dear. Was nothing what it seemed? How stupid was I?

I kept thinking, *I cannot believe this is my life.* And it was. It was my life.

Every day, I went through the motions. I packed lunches. I got dressed. I put on make-up. I smiled. I volunteered. I laughed with my friends, but it felt like a fun-house version of my life. You know how when you are watching a horror movie and the scene is idyllic, it usually means something terrifying is about to happen? That's what it felt like, as though the soundtrack to my life was that super creepy music that all ice cream trucks are apparently mandated to play. A distant, tinny, haunting version of what it used to be.

In the face of all that heaviness, I began to lose weight. That felt right, too. I felt untethered, as though at any moment I could fly off the face of the earth. The things that had grounded me in my life were gone. Or broken. Either way, weightlessness felt right.

I started doing two things consistently - drinking every evening and not eating every day.

What I did not do was tell anyone the truth. No one. Not my sisters, not my best friend.

Eventually, people began to notice my weight. I stepped out of the shower one morning, and my husband said, *You look great*. I felt a wave of fury wash over me. That was beginning of it. That was when my not eating became intentional. When I began actively not eating. I think on some level I wanted to look outwardly the way I felt inwardly. Wrecked.

You know that scene in Madagascar with the penguins?

"Smile and wave, boys. Smile and wave."

That was me. Every day. I'd put on my ever-shrinking jeans and plaster my face in more and more makeup. I'd pretend I didn't notice how much hair came out in my hands each morning when I showered. The worse it got inside, the 'better' I looked outside.

After the first ten pounds, friends and acquaintances began to say things. When I'd lost twenty, it became a daily occurrence. Every day, I would hear how great I looked. *You look amazing!* and, *What are you doing?* I would always say, *Atkins.* I felt shame about that for a long time. For anyone who was trying to lose weight in a healthy way, it must have been discouraging to see the weight falling off of me, seemingly without a struggle.

But it was a struggle- just not the right kind.

The last time I got on the scale I weighed 103 lbs. That did not get me to stop starving myself, though. I did, however, stop getting on the scale.

And I got smaller still.

All told, I lost almost fifty pounds in seven months. And I have never gotten so much positive feedback in my life. And mostly from other women.

And I knew it wasn't true. I didn't look great. I was disappearing, bit by bit, every single day. The only two consistent exceptions were my friends, Angela and Juleen. Juleen said on several occasions, *You look beautiful, but are you eating?* I would reassure her that I was, but we both knew I was lying.

Angela, my best friend, my chosen sister, lived next door to me. Our houses were connected by a pretty little path through the woods. I remember going over to her house one night and turning back halfway because my size two jeans were falling down and I knew it would worry her. She was already worried sick about me. I am so sorry to have done that to her.

I was living two existences. At home, when the kids were at school, I was, quite literally, on the floor. Undone. Wasting away, every day. And then there was the shiny, happy version. I had cute clothes and I smiled and I was in the PTA. And I was the 'right' size.

You know how actors will pick up an empty prop suitcase and pretend it's heavy? I did the opposite. I am really, really good at 'fine.' Like, the best. Most of the world would very much prefer you be that way, you know. I wasn't telling my story - I was selling one, though. I carried around so many heavy secrets and pretended they weighed nothing, I was presenting a polished up, highly edited version of a life I wasn't really living.

You know what they say, though, practice makes perfect. I'd been honing my story-selling skills for decades.

I had a really lovely email from a woman in my old neighborhood, not a close friend, but someone I knew casually and liked. She expressed her sorrow at the news of my divorce and said something along the lines of having seen me living in that beautiful yellow house, walking hand in hand with my kid to school every day, and thinking she knew what my life was. She told me how sad it made her to think how much pain I'd been in. That email meant the world to me. It's so true. We decide about one another based on jean size and wardrobe and granite countertops. We decide about each other from the outside. In other words, based on exactly nothing. It's so much more comfortable not to look behind the curtain.

As women, we get rewarded for being the smallest possible versions of ourselves in every way. Be nice, be quiet, be THIN. I had become the absolute tiniest version of me. I'd become terrified and disillusioned and exhausted, and I was keeping more and more secrets.

Yes, I've eaten.
Sure, I slept.
Only one glass.
He's traveling.
I'm fine.
We're fine.

"I was so wary then
The ugly American
Thinner than oxygen
Tough as a whore
I said you can lie to me
I own what's inside of me
And nothing surprises me anymore"

Shawn Colvin

That was me. I was thinner than the air I kept forgetting to breathe. And even though I felt awful, there was a sort of power in it, too. It was the only thing I could seem to control. I got more positive attention for my appearance then than at any other point in my life. And I was dying. I really was.

My reasons for not telling the truth of what my life had become were myriad and complex.

First, I was ashamed. Deeply ashamed that I was valued so little, that the life I'd carefully built was a house of cards. I was ashamed for all the reasons women blame themselves when marriages collapse - I wasn't enough, I was boring, I was getting older, I'd gained weight, and then, of course, the main support beam in the house of story I'd built, the load bearing wall, the belief that there was something inherently wrong with me. That I was unworthy, unlovable.

It didn't take a lot for me to get to a place of shame. Shame's a pretty cozy spot for me.

I was also desperate to make my marriage work. To save it, somehow. If I just tried harder, got thinner, dusted every surface, said yes to every nolt...

I couldn't say it out loud. If I said it out loud it would be real. If I saw the shock and anger and judgment on my friends' and sisters' faces, I'd have to integrate it It would always be a part of our story moving forward. I would be exposed.

I also knew how I'd reacted when people I loved went through something similar. I knew the rage I felt, the way I'd internalized their pain. I remembered my frustration that they didn't just leave, which is what I always said I would do. I knew it. I knew exactly what I would do in that situation until I was in that situation. Everything is different, close up.

I was afraid of being told I should go. I was afraid to be judged. I was afraid people would think I was pathetic for staying - for even wanting to stay.

So I said nothing. I smiled and I joked with friends. I powered through my hangovers and worked out frantically twice a day and I didn't say a word to anyone.

I kept the secret as though my life depended on it because the life I knew and loved did, in fact, depend on it.

I kept the secret because I have always been a secret keeper. I kept the secret because I knew from experience that speaking the truth was a sure-fire way to lose your family.

Eventually, there was no choice but to tell. No amount of denial or hustle was going to save a marriage that was fundamentally broken. And I now realize it was broken long before the events that were to be its death knell. It would be years after my divorce before I truly came back to life, before I stopped trying to disappear.

It would take crashing and burning at rock bottom before I would tell the rest of my story and allow myself to be fully seen.

CHAPTER 8

The Fault in my Scars

"On the girl's brown legs there were
many small white scars.
I was thinking, do those scars cover the whole of you,
like the stars and the moons on your dress?
I thought that would be pretty too,
and I ask you right here please to agree with me that a
scar is never ugly.
That is what the scar makers want us to think.
But you and I, we must make an agreement
to defy them.
We must see all scars as beauty. Okay?
This will be our secret.
Because take it from me, a scar does not
form on the dying.
A scar means,
I survived."

Chris Cleave

THERE IS A scene in Good Will Hunting where Robin Williams' character, Sean Maguire, has Will cornered and he has his social services file in his hand. They talk about the abuse Will suffered as a boy, and Sean starts saying, *It's not your fault.* Over and over again.

Yeah, I know.

It's not your fault, Sean repeats.

Will half laughs.

It's not your fault.

Will becomes angry.

It's not your fault.

Will begins sobbing.

Me too.

I've probably seen that movie ten times and that scene always affects me the same way. Part of the reason is that it is a beautifully written, gorgeously acted scene. I'm sure most people watching it are moved.

I'm not moved. I just recognize the terrain.

There is a chasm between the brain and the heart, a chasm so deep, so wide, so profound, that for some it is impossible to traverse. The brain can know something is logically, unimpeachably true, and the heart may never accept it. It's the difference between facts and feelings, knowing and believing.

I am a survivor of sexual abuse.

That's something that until recently I'd never said out loud. Survivor, that is. I've said I was sexually abused. I've said I was a victim of abuse. I've become more and more open about it in the last few years. Never used the word survivor, though - not even when it became the empowered thing to say. Not even when OPRAH said it.

I think that is because for much of the more than three and a half decades since it happened I knew the jury was still out on whether or not I would survive it. We don't all, you know? We don't all survive.

I am a survivor of sexual abuse.

It was not my fault.

I was a little girl. He was a grown man.

It was not my fault.

I know that. Of course, I know that.

The thing about shame is that it doesn't so much live in your brain, as it inhabits your heart. It is a parasite that takes up lodging in your soul. I have been host to my shame for so long that it had become hard to imagine my life without it.

Shame was always my baseline. Shame always felt a lot like home to me.

What's so deeply insidious about that particular type of abuse is that it fundamentally changes how a child feels about who they are, how they see the world, and how they believe the world sees them.

I used to think everyone knew. In fact, I used to think they could smell it on me. Literally. I was obviously bad. I was the type of girl boys wanted, but not for their girlfriend. I never thought I was beautiful, but I always knew I had that thing - whatever it is. That's another thing about shame - you wear it. Every day. You just assume it's visible.

Maybe it is.

I can look back and see how my abuse informed the decisions I made in my life. The people I chose, the power I gave them.

It's really just in the past few years that I've decided I don't want to live that way anymore. It's another way in which the implosion of my marriage was a gift. You know how on home renovation shows when they are touring a disaster of a house they say need to take it down to the studs? Total gut job?

Maybe that was me. Maybe I was a gut job. I'd been trying to do cosmetic repairs for years. Prettying up the outside stuff, when really I needed to strip it all away. Down to the bones. That's what my divorce did for me. It took away the 'perfect' and left me with the mess. My very own ground zero.

A while back I decided to write my abuser a letter. He's dead - passed away years ago. Doesn't matter — it's to the version of him that lives within me, anyway.

To the Thief,

If I were to list what you stole from me, I would write forever.

I've heard other survivors say that their childhood was stolen. I suppose that's close to being true for me. What you stole was the child within me. I was an ancient ruin before I was ten.

When I look at school pictures after that summer they look like me… almost. It's as though it's a very realistic mask of the girl I used to be. But blank. Like a light went out. I turned the corners of my mouth up for the camera because I was an obedient girl and I knew that's what was expected of me - but there was no joy. I was guessing at normal.

I looked tired.

I was tired. All the time.

You stole my belief that I was safe in the world. Even in my little world. Once you know what people are capable of- the evil that is possible - you never feel entirely safe again. When someone who is supposed to love you, supposed to protect you, violates your trust and desecrates your body - you feel as though danger lurks everywhere. If you aren't safe in the cocoon of your own family, you come to believe you will never be safe anywhere. Ever.

You took from me my sense of self. I didn't get the opportunity to form a strong identity before having my sexuality be the way I defined who I was. I don't remember a time when that wasn't the way I viewed my worth. I knew that's where my value lay because that's what you taught me. You didn't hone in on me for my intelligence, or my kindness, or my personality. You wanted to dominate and punish me. To inhabit and destroy me. You taught me to hate my body. I still have not entirely unlearned that lesson, even more than three decades later.

For a long time, I carried around so much anger. I disguised it as sarcasm and cleverness, but frequently I was just mean and defensive. I nurtured a small seed of hatred in my heart that bore your name, and it informed the decisions I made, the people I brought into my life and the woman I became.

I know I cannot have peace or true happiness by continuing to do that. If my focus is on the wounds of the past, I will miss out on the blessings of the future- and I am unwilling to allow that. In order to cast out that darkness, in order to banish that hatred, what I finally realize is that I need to forgive you.

As inconceivable as that seems, I know in my heart it is the only way.

I don't want to carry these heavy things anymore. Without forgiveness, there is no freedom from this. From you. And I want to travel light.

What I know for sure is that monsters like you are not born, they are carefully crafted. As I am your creation, you were someone's handiwork as well.

Someone stole your light. Someone killed the boy within you, the same way you murdered the little girl within me, I am certain of it. You turned it outward, and I tried to destroy myself from within. My continued mistreatment was an inside job.

I mourn for the boy you once were, for your lost innocence. For what you might have been. Nobody, not even you, is all one thing. I am sure you had gifts and talents. I know you came into this world good. The only thing I remember about you is what you did to me, but I am sure that is not the totality of who you were.

I mourn for your other victims - the ones I know about and the ones who remain anonymous. My nameless, faceless, shattered sisters.

I am going to do my best to let you go. To have this be one thing that happened to me a very long time ago. Not the defining thing. Not the totality of who I am and who I hope to become. Just a chapter in the book of my life - perhaps never completely closed, but whose pages I hope to revisit less and less. There is too much happiness ahead of me. There is too much goodness and grace in the world to spend time reliving such pain.

I refuse to continue to be your host. I will not feed you anymore. You own a great deal of my past, but I will give you none of my future.

You cannot have that.

It's time to sit in the sun.

Goodbye.

Laura

CHAPTER 9

He Wrote it Down

*"Some things cannot be fixed; they can
only be carried."*

Megan Devine

MY BEAUTIFUL COUSIN, who I'd not seen in 35 years, and I set out
to dance on our grandfather's grave.

Our first dilemma was, of course, song choice. You have to
have the right song. We bandied a few song titles about. Alanis
Morrisette was a front-runner.

Obviously.

We drove to the town where he lived, and where he is bur-
ied. We drove to the town where we were abused. Driving down
the picturesque New England roads, I felt a little faint. Mary
felt a little barfy. We pulled into a store parking lot and Mary
spent some quality time behind a dumpster, hurling. It happens.

We weren't entirely sure where the cemetery was, so we
pulled into a police station to ask for directions. I said, jokingly,
We should go in and file a police report. Mary said, *What would happen
if we went inside and filed a police report?*

I said, *Let's do it.*

We walked in, after Mary barfed again, and there was a darling older police officer behind the glass window. Mary told him we were looking for the cemetery and I had a moment of thinking we probably weren't really going to do it. Then my beautiful cousin, who is the bravest person I know, said, *And we would like to report a crime.*

That got his attention.

She said, *Our grandfather sexually molested us 35 years ago, and we want to report him.*

We were ushered into a conference room and a young officer came in to talk to us. He handles all of their sexual assault and rape cases. He introduced himself, sat down and proceeded to ask us questions about what happened. Names, addresses, dates. I called my sister and put her on speakerphone. We were all crying.

Sweetie, I said, He's writing it down.

He wrote it down.

We said, *This happened to us*, and he listened. He WROTE IT DOWN.

I cannot begin to tell you how powerful that was.

He said several times, *I don't want to open any wounds, so if you don't want to answer this, that's okay.* Finally, I said, *The wounds are all still open. Obviously. What do you want to know?*

I found myself saying, to a police officer, *I was raped.*

I never thought that would happen.

Then Mary asked a question I would not have thought to ask, but the answer to which I really needed. She said, *What would have happened to him if someone had reported it?* The officer told us the procedural things, he said he would have interviewed us, he would have interviewed our grandfather, he would have corroborated what he could. And then, he said-

I would have driven down the street and arrested him.

That is what should have happened.

We know there is nothing to be done. We know there will be no consequences, and no justice. Life is staggeringly unfair, sometimes.

But there is a record. We walked into that police station holding the jagged shards of our story, of our childhood, and said, *LOOK. THIS HAPPENED.* And Officer Paul Smith bore witness. He wrote it down.

In few days, the police report will be available and Mary will go get three copies. Or, if she makes good on her threat to send it out in lieu of a Christmas card next year, maybe many more. But at least three. We will each have a copy.

We asked Officer Smith if anyone else ever comes forward about our grandfather- because we know with absolute certainty there are other victims - to please give them our information. We want to meet them.

At that point, we thought we were still going to go to the cemetery. Officer Paul offered us a police escort.

I think it is important to note, in the face of so much awfulness, that people really are mostly very good. He was so kind. He took it so seriously. He honored our loss.

Mary decided she's not quite ready to dance on his grave. That's okay. We've found each other again.

We've got nothing but time.

That's where this was supposed to end.

Then I got a call this morning, from Officer Paul.

He said, *Can you come in? I have something I want to tell you guys.*

So.

Mary and I just got back. We were at the police station for hours. Talking to a mama about her daughter. She told us what happened. She told us what our grandfather did to her girl. We bore witness for her. Officer Paul wrote it down.

Guys, I don't quite know what to do with any of this. It's a LOT. I have a crushing headache, and Mary and I have made an agreement that we will spend the rest of the night talking about Adam Levine's abs. That's it. That's all we've got. But, my world is lighter than it was yesterday.

CHAPTER 10

White Flag

"When I find myself in times of trouble,
Mother Mary comes to me,
speaking words of wisdom,
Let it Be.
And in my hour of darkness,
She is standing right in front of me,
speaking words of wisdom,
Let it Be."

Paul McCartney

BEFORE I PUBLISHED The Fault in my Scars, I sent it to my friend Glennon to read. Glennon is brilliant, funny, and wise, and a brave and vulnerable writer. She is a big part of why I began writing again. I love her.

She said this:

The essay felt like a holy surrender. Like a long-awaited surrender to the truth of things - like a giving up of the horrible, backbreaking mis-belief that your past could have been any different.

It was a glory filled holding up of your arms to the air with a
shout: HERE I AM! LET IT BE!
Everything beautiful comes now.
After surrender.
You know that.

I have been thinking a LOT about her words.

I used to hate the expression, 'It is what it is.' It always smacked of defeatism to me. I see it differently now. It might have something to do with saying the Serenity Prayer 947 times a day.

I was sexually abused. That is a fact and facts are not negotiable.

I spent so much time trying to change my past. As though I could will myself into having had a different, better, safer, childhood.

You hear people say all the time that we get dealt a hand in life. That simply isn't true. We get dealt MANY hands. Different hands at different stages of life. Different cards for different seasons.

My cousin and I, we got dealt a lousy hand early in life. A terrible, dark, painful, hand. Judging by the number of comments, messages, and emails I've received after publishing He Wrote It Down, an awful lot of you did too.

"And when the broken hearted people
living in the world agree,

> There will be an answer,
> Let it Be.
> For though they may be parted,
> there is still a chance that they will see,
> There will be answer,
> Let it Be."

But we have all been dealt many hands since then. Some good, some bad. We have, each time, the choice to play them or not. *Know when to hold 'em, know when to fold 'em* – amiright Kenny?

The problem for me, and I think for a lot of survivors of childhood abuse, sexual or otherwise, is that we spend the rest of our lives trying to play that one hand. Again and again. Perhaps hoping for a different outcome, perhaps hoping that the cards themselves will change.

The thing is, if you keep playing those cards, you'll likely find yourself reliving the trauma over and over as well. It might look a little different, the main characters might have different faces, the circumstances might not be exactly the same, but you will find yourself feeling the same way, repeating the same patterns. I did.

But friends, that hand is over. Those cards are gone. And everyone else has moved on, has been dealt new cards and is playing them. We get stuck, though, because we are still trying desperately for a different past. We clutch those cards with the unyielding grasp of a child, still trying to win a game that has long ended. Fighting against the truth of what happened. Maybe if I'd done this or that. Maybe if someone had believed me. We are trying to re-negotiate things that have already happened and that never, never works.

I can guarantee this: if you do not accept your past, it will never be over. Ever.

I wish things had been different for my cousin and me. I so wish things could have been different for all of the brave women and men who have entrusted me with their stories. Thousands of you bravely shared stories of violence, pain, and betrayal. I read every single one. I wrote down every single name. I wish each of you'd had what we all deserve: a childhood devoid of abuse. Everyone should have a childhood that is carefree, nurturing, safe, and full of wonder; protected by those entrusted with their care.

Those are simply not the cards we were dealt.

No amount of wishing will do a damned thing. No amount of shaking my fist at the sky can undo what was done, can return what was lost.

I think we get stuck with acceptance and surrender the same way we do with forgiveness. We think if we forgive, that means the people who harmed us get a pass, somehow. That what they did was okay. That we're okay. We think of acceptance as a stamp of approval on what happened. We've been taught to equate surrender with quitting and losing.

You know that moment in so many boxing movies, when the guy is on the ground, bleeding? He's taken too many blows to the head and he's been beaten unrecognizable. There comes a moment when even the people who wanted him to win are shouting, *STAY DOWN*. He keeps trying to get up and the guys in his corner are like, *DUDE. You're gonna DIE.*

It's not about losing at that point - it's that he cannot win. I think surrender is giving yourself over to things you cannot change. I think surrender happens when you stop fighting the unwinnable battle.

We survivors spend a lot of time and energy shadow boxing opponents long gone. It's exhausting and we cannot, will not, ever win.

We have limited resources as human beings, and if we use them up fighting battles we cannot win, we are tacitly agreeing not to fight the ones we can.

I think that is one reason why there was so much power in the writing down of our story and in Officer Paul taking down his report. It was not a defeat, it was a victorious surrender. It's why, when I shared the blog, I said simply, *Friends, here's what happened.*

It's what happened. I give. I can stop fighting the fact of it, and decide what to do with the gifts that horrible part of my life gave me, because there truly are always gifts.

I am gearing up for some battles that need fighting. I want to fight some battles I can win.

"And when the night is cloudy,
there is still a light that shines on me.
Shine on until tomorrow,
Let it Be.
I wake up to the sound of music,
Mother Mary comes to me,
Speaking words of wisdom,
Let it Be."

I am waking up to the sound of music now. Every day. I have music in my heart again, because I folded that hand. It played out the way it played out. Those were my cards. I am ready for some new ones.

Everything beautiful comes now.

CHAPTER 11

Civil War

"That's the thing about pain. It demands to be felt."

John Green

I HAVE ALWAYS hated my body.

I can name twenty things off the top of my head that I wish I could change - I wouldn't even need to think about it. I hate my elbows. Who hates their elbows, for heaven's sake? It is hard for me to accept compliments gracefully. I immediately want to deflect, or make a joke, or tell you the many things that are wrong with me.

Some of that is just the world in which we live. You don't need to have experienced sexual trauma as a girl to be awash in self-loathing as a grown woman. We are bombarded with unrealistic beauty ideals and the constant repetitive beat of, *you are not enough, you are not enough, you are not enough.*

As a survivor of sexual abuse, those beats frequently fall in time with the rhythmic story you tell yourself, *I am bad, I am bad, I am bad.*

Those beats? They are the drums of war.

I've waged war against my body for as long as I can remember. Hate is a strong word, an ugly word, but it's what I felt for my physical being for as long as I can remember. Hate.

I have had many conversations with people, women mostly, about the ways in which sexual abuse affects you long term. I think it is astounding, the ways we find to survive.

Some of us block out the memories. Our young brains determine that the trauma is too much to handle and they bury the truth. The mind compartmentalizes the memory. It puts the pain on layaway. You pay a tiny bit, over a long period of time, but eventually, the balance comes due. With interest.

The pain demands to be felt.

So many of us battle with weight. Some gain pounds as a type of armor, a way to keep people at arms' length in an attempt to protect ourselves, a way to stay safe. Some deny themselves food, some purge. Some of us try to disappear. Literally. I did. I tried to disappear.

So many of us anesthetize, with food, or alcohol, or drugs, or sex - all in ways that are harmful to our bodies. Temporary fixes at best. Treacherous band-aids. But still, eventually, the pain demands to be felt.

I had several women share their shame and guilt over their promiscuity. I had one woman tell me it was proof she had invited her abuse. If she really was traumatized why would she seek out sex? I can only speak to my experience, but when you are taught at a very young age that no doesn't mean no and that you do not have ultimate dominion over your own body, you believe it. When you are taught that your value lies solely in your sexual being, you believe it. Some are seeking to reclaim their sexual power, or are chasing the temporary pleasure to stave off the crushing pain, pain that *demands* to be felt.

I think the mind and the body are miraculous. I think we subconsciously find ways to survive. When the body undergoes severe physical trauma it goes into shock. Systems slow and shut down. You are protected from the pain because it is simply too much to bear. The same is true of emotional trauma.

Your brain finds ways to protect you. But just like with physical shock, you cannot live indefinitely in that state. The very things you are doing to protect yourself from the pain will eventually kill you. You need to come out of shock at some point. As Robert Frost said, *the only way 'round is through.*

To come out the other side, to feel the sun on your face again, you need to feel the pain. It is unspeakably hard to sign up for that. To know it's coming and to stay still for it. To not find ways to numb yourself. It takes a staggering amount of bravery.

I am finally forgiving myself for the things that I did to survive. Those things that seemed foolish or harmful from the cheap seats. Those things that seemed self-destructive and counter-intuitive from the outside. Many of them were, honestly, but I'm not sure I could have survived the pain earlier. I think they were desperate measures, but then, that's what's called for in desperate times.

I am extending the olive branch to younger me. I'm calling a truce and laying down my arms. I am going to stop blaming my body, and I am going to stop shaming my brain.

No one gets to judge how you managed to survive, friends. No one. No one gets to shame you for whatever you did to get yourself to the place where you can live through feeling the pain. Not even you.

You survived, honey. Not everyone does, you know.

You miraculous girl. You miraculous boy. You clever, resilient child, you.

You can stop hurting yourself. You can shed your armor and still be safe.

You can be seen and still be safe. You are so much stronger than you give yourself credit for. You are being held hostage. Meet the demands. Feel the pain. It will take some courage, but we already know how brave you are. You are so, so brave.

You are strong enough to walk through the pain and into the sunlight - I promise you. Freedom is just around the bend.

CHAPTER 12

The Choices We Make

"He loved her, of course, but better than that, he chose
her day after day.
Choice: that was the thing."

Sherman Alexie

I'M NOT CERTAIN how old I was. I was little, though - maybe four? It was winter in Massachusetts. It was an overcast day and the snow was piled high. My family lived in an apartment complex at the time and I was playing outside in the parking lot. I was scrambling up a snow bank created when the parking lot was plowed. This was many years ago, back in the days when children were allowed to climb.

I slipped and my leg slid down the icy drift and became wedged between the snow bank and the front bumper of a car. I was wearing one of those gargantuan one-piece A Christmas Story-style snowsuits and thick winter boots, and there was no freeing myself.

I remember being terrified that my leg was broken and I would be stuck there forever. I remember thinking I might die.

I've always been a little on the dramatic side.

Now I'm sure my parents weren't too far away, though this was the seventies, so who knows? In any case, in due time (and probably much more quickly than it seemed to me in my panicked state) my father came. I remember him wiping my tears with his snowy gloves, which only served to make my whole face wetter but somehow helped anyway.

He hovered over me, using his always logical, engineer brain to carefully extricate me from my icy little prison without injuring me. I vividly recall looking up into his handsome face. He scowled in concentration as he repositioned my leg to slide it out and I thought for an instant he was angry with me. Then, once I was freed, his brow relaxed and he kissed me on the forehead.

I was completely unharmed. I don't remember this moment because it was particularly traumatic or because I was hurt. I remember this moment because I felt safe.

⚬

You know what the best thing was about being proposed to? It wasn't the ring. It wasn't any grand gesture, certainly. It was being proven wrong. I never thought anyone would ask me to marry him.

It was knowing someone chose me. It was a new experience and one that made me feel safe.

When my marriage ended, I felt forsaken. Un-chosen. In my darkest moments of feeling that way, I thought, *Of course. Of course, this happened. This was always going to happen. This is what men do.* When you feel worthless, it sort of makes sense when people tell you they don't love you. When they throw you away.

It's painful, but then, that's what you do with disposable things, isn't it?

When I told the truth about my abuse my mother believed me and my father did not. They were going through an ugly divorce. There was a tremendous amount of anger. My abuse became part of that narrative when it was, in fact, completely unrelated.

I remember sitting in that family counseling session and feeling my dad's anger wash over me. I had obviously done something very wrong. I completely internalized it. I felt as though I was folding in on myself, getting smaller and smaller as I sat there. The origami girl.

If I could have taken it back I would have, right then and there. That's the thing about the truth, though, it's a bell you can't un-ring.

And then, incrementally, he was pretty much gone from our lives. We saw him less and less frequently. Our father was farther and farther away.

I remember the first time I saw a trailer for Taken. I remember being moved to tears by the notion of a father who would go to any lengths to rescue his daughter. The righteous anger of a protector.

Freakin' Liam Neeson.

As a young girl, when your father walks away from you, when he deserts you when things get hard and you need him the most, maybe you begin to unconsciously repeat that pattern. Perhaps you attract men who will do the same thing. It's familiar. Comfortable, even.

I think that factors hugely into my struggles with faith. Actually, I think it is *the* struggle I've had with my faith.

We refer to God as our Father.

We are told He loves us unconditionally, and never, ever leaves us.

It took me a very long time to be able to reconcile those things.

I remember listening to a pastor at my church give a sermon about how our earthly fathers can let us down, but our Heavenly Father never will. I always struggled with believing that, with trusting that God had a plan and would be there for me. That He would never leave, no matter what.

In my personal experience, fathers and unconditional love are mutually exclusive things. Fortunately, elsewhere in my life, I know many amazing fathers. I had an uncle who was very much a father figure to me, and the father of my best friend growing up was always there for me. I had older male cousins who were very protective of me.

I'm blessed, really. It's an embarrassment of riches.

When my son was about six months old, I took him to meet my dad. We had a conversation in which he told me he didn't believe me about the abuse when I was young but that he did now. It seemed as though he felt he was offering me a gift or doing me a favor. Maybe I was supposed to thank him? Perhaps he wanted a relationship with his grandson and he thought saying that was the cost of doing business. I don't suppose I'll ever know.

I thought and thought about it that night, about what that should have meant to me. About what it *would* have meant to me if it were true. I lay awake with my baby son in my arms and my abuser smiling at me from a framed photograph opposite the bed where we lay.

There is no universe in which, if someone violated my child that way, I would have a photo of them in my house much less in the room where they were staying. Where they were expected to sleep.

I remember seeing the movie Awakenings starring Robin Williams and Robert DeNiro, and being struck how once Robin Williams grew that beard he looked exactly like my dad. There's a scene in the movie where his character is wearing a short-sleeved button down plaid shirt – the very kind my dad favored. The resemblance was uncanny.

From that time on I felt such a connection to Robin. It was one of his great gifts as an actor, that as a big a star as he was you sort of felt as though you knew him. He became a bit of a father figure to me in some ways. When he died I was heartbroken.

I've spent most of my life being heartbroken about my dad. I've grieved the loss of him since I was a tiny, little girl. He's still around - well, as much as he's ever been.

If I met him today, if there weren't all of these dark and heavy things between us, I like to think we would be great friends. He's funny and charming and handsome. He's smart. He's really generous of spirit with the people in his life.

I just don't happen to be one of them.

I've finally accepted that. It is a loss and one that I have mourned deeply. It is an ache that I carry with me every day. But having a relationship with me would either require him to truly acknowledge things he cannot or will not, or it would require me to keep my pain, my inconvenient truths in the dark where they would eat me alive. It would require me to remain a secret-keeper, to fold in on myself. It would require me to take the sharp corners of my anger and fold them down, to take the corners that are my truth and make them a wing or a petal. Something pleasing – a flower or a swan. Something nicer to look at. *That corner over there - the truth of our family? Let's bend that down. There. That's better. Prettier.*

I did that for a very long time, but not one minute more.

I do not hate my dad. I never have. I love him, actually. I just love me more.

I spent time with my dad a few years back packing up my sister's house after her husband died. It was a hard time. Awful. We worked really well together, though. There were a couple of times when he marveled at some trait we shared or the similar way we approached things. It was touching in a sad sort of way. I'm in my forties and it was a revelation to him that I was his girl. In so many ways, I am. I am very much his girl.

CHAPTER 13

Comfort and Joy

"What kills a soul? Exhaustion, secret keeping, image management. And what brings a soul back from the dead? Honesty, connection, grace."

Shauna Niequist

WHEN I WAS twenty-one, I found myself sitting in the hallway of the maternity ward, waiting on Barbara Bush to get her act together. The then First Lady was touring the hospital and no one was being allowed to leave until the tour was over. My son was the world's cutest hostage in the nursery and I was stuck in the hallway in a wheelchair, alone with my thoughts.

That was not optimal.

I was terrified. I had this fear they would bring the wrong baby to me and I wouldn't know the difference. I was worried about the car seat. I wasn't confident I'd installed it properly. I was so tired. I'd gotten a five-minute lesson in diaper changing and umbilical cord care, and they'd given me a pamphlet on breast-feeding - and now they were prepared to entrust me with keeping another person alive. What could go wrong? I thought, *This cannot be the actual way things work, can it? This is utterly irresponsible.*

Mrs. Bush gave me plenty of time to question the judgment of professionals who seemed inclined to let me leave the hospital with a tiny, fragile human.

I lived with my mom and my sister at that point, and people kept saying things about how my son would have two moms, three moms. I am certain they were intended as supportive comments, but that's not how they *felt*. They felt like a lack of belief in my ability to handle it on my own. They felt like attempts to undermine my role as his actual mother. I became determined to not need help. To do everything myself, and make it seem easy even when it was so, so hard, because even the admission of struggle seemed like a failure to me. I felt as though if I admitted how hard I found motherhood sometimes it would validate every fear, every doubt - theirs and mine. I need to get this motherhood thing right. I needed to do it perfectly. He deserved that. I wanted to give that, to be that for him.

⟶⟦◉ ◉⟧⟵

I have always been a worker. I might not have always been the smartest person in the room, but I'd out-hustle you, bank on it. I always prided myself on my work ethic and my desire to do things well.

I believe that all perfectionism is rooted in *not enough* - a belief that *I don't do enough*. When you factor in shame that becomes, *I am not enough, I cannot be enough.* I think when you believe in your inherent worth you don't spend your whole life trying to prove it.

Women get rewarded for such weird things.

Being small. Being busy. Being exhausted. Being selfless.

How many times have you heard someone say as an accolade, *She never thinks of herself.* And we all nod and acknowledge she's a saint.

Well, you know how most saints get that coveted moniker? Martyrdom.

Yaaaaaaaay.

Part of the practice of sobriety is examining your character traits and behavior. Once you've inventoried your stuff, you begin to see patterns emerge. Control, fear, dishonesty...

It's interesting how words can change. Well, I suppose the words themselves don't change, but their meaning, impact - even the reaction they provoke in us does, depending on where we are in our lives.

Before I got sober I would have put perfectionism and busyness firmly in my asset column. I wore exhaustion like a badge of honor. I thought my inability to relax or unapologetically take time for myself was a good thing.

I thought these traits were part of being a good mother. I actually thought they were a necessary component of motherhood, if you were doing it right. And I know I am not alone in that. Check in at any school bus stop or PTA meeting and see how many women are trying to out-stress, out-busy, out-fatigue, or out-suffer one another. Watch just about any family sitcom. If there's a character of a mom pay attention to how she is written. I'm willing to bet she's exasperated, beleaguered, un-helped, and worn out.

My perfectionism was very much rooted in my desire for other people to not see me for who I believed myself to truly be. I wanted to be perceived as having it together, doing it all. There was no greater stage for this insanity than my parenting. I desperately wanted to be a good mother. I wanted to give my kids the childhood I wanted to have had; safe, orderly, magical, innocent. I wanted to do it RIGHT.

When you are invested in one way being the only right way that does not make for a lot of fun and it doesn't allow for col-laboration or mistakes – your own or other people's. It leaves precious little room for grace. If I found it hard to relax, I can only imagine how it difficult it was for the people around me. I was so rigid and so concerned about how things appeared and how they needed to be done. That doesn't leave much room for ease or for happiness.

I loved coming up with family traditions, which can be great and meaningful and fun, but then I enforced them like a mafia henchman. The house had to be spotless, which is pretty but not comfortable. Birthday parties had to be perfect but ap-pear to have been thrown together effortlessly. The holidays had to seem magical, which, I guarantee, meant they were not. You can't mandate joy.

I used to spend so much time focused on making each Christmas the best Christmas ever. Last Christmas was a stan-dard to be exceeded- this year needed to be *even better*. It was gluttony, really. It was a gluttonous approach to joy, and any time you see someone indulging in gluttony it comes from a fear of scarcity - count on it. I was behaving as though joy was a finite resource to be scavenged and hoarded.

It was all hustle, and hustle is the farthest thing from self-worth. Hustle is, *If I don't make myself the linchpin of this whole operation, there won't be room for me at the table.* Hustle is, *If I'm not indispensable then I don't have worth.* It's so insidious, because it's such self-centered behavior masquerading as selflessness.

The need to be necessary is backbreaking and soul-depleting. And it's a vicious circle. People stroke your ego and tell you how X, Y, and Z would quite simply *not happen* were it not for your efforts. I used to think that was a strength, being that crucial. Now I know it's selfish. If I truly care about a project, an event, any endeavor, really, I should want there to be a deeper bench. I should welcome help. Otherwise it's ego and fear - which is a little redundant, when I think about it.

I imagine it was difficult to be my child during those times. Actually, I know it was. You cannot put that much pressure on yourself without imparting to your kids the notion that doing so is good. And when I was setting an alarm for 4:00 a.m. on Christmas morning not only so I could have baked, lit candles, turned on the tree and the Christmas music, done my makeup and popped the champagne cork (because, obv.) but also, and this is just unseemly, so everyone knew it. *Look how much I did. Look how much I give.*

That puts so much pressure on other people to enjoy it enough, appreciate it enough. The weight of that expectation is crushing.

I remember one year one of the kids had a pirate party for their birthday. I organized a treasure hunt that involved me writing ten clues in verse for a scavenger hunt and then actually burying treasure in the backyard. With a shovel. Like a lunatic.

When party guests exclaimed over how much work it must have been I am sure I gave the impression I did it in my sleep, and I am also sure I was a wreck leading up to the party. Probably less than delightful and present for my kid's big day.

I cared deeply that strangers believe it all came easily to me and that my near and dear knew how hard it was. My God, that's jacked up.

That kind of perfectionism is a form of secret keeping, even if the only secret is that you are fully human and flawed and that life is hard. Now, that might be the worst kept secret in the world, but the thing about secrets is this – the intention to keep the secret matters, even if you're unsuccessful. The intention to not be seen is still there even if you are hiding in plain sight. The need to control people's perception of you is always rooted in fear and it is always dishonest.

It's such a painful realization to come to that you can love your family so much and still not love them very well.

I am grateful to have the opportunity to live differently, now. Sometimes I see glimpses of the patterns I instilled by way of example in my kids and I feel a flash of fear because I want better for them. I want them to know they were born enough. They came into this world so incredibly loved and necessary and ENOUGH. I worry that they'll fall prey to hustle and perfectionism the way I did *because* I did.

Holidays are very different, today. People get up when they want to get up. As it turns out, we don't all have to enjoy things the same way. My way is not the right way, it's just my way. And I know my people would rather have me rested and present and sober than the way I used to be. They'd rather have Christmas be good enough than look perfect. I would rather be loved for the flawed, weird, imperfect person that I am than be admired for trying to be something I am not. That feels like progress.

CHAPTER 14

Allow Me to Introduce Myself

"But you can't get to any of these truths by sitting in a field smiling beatifically, avoiding your anger and damage and grief. Your anger and damage and grief are the way to the truth. We don't have much truth to express unless we have gone into those rooms and closets and woods and abysses that we were told not go in to. When we have gone in and looked around for a long while, just breathing and finally taking it in — then we will be able to speak in our own voice and to stay in the present moment. And that moment is home."

Anne Lamott

WE ALL HAVE things we don't want to look at.

Not looking at something might seem like a passive thing, and I suppose sometimes it is. Sometimes we have something in our lives that we've not examined because it simply has not occurred to us to do so. In those instances, it is usually because whatever the thing is, it isn't a big enough concern to be on our radar.

That isn't me. I am a fairly reflective person by nature. Given that I am wired that way, if I am not examining something in my life it is likely intentional. I tell you, friends, I can make not looking at something an active pursuit. Practically an aerobic activity. You could burn calories with the way I avoid looking at things I do not want to see.

There is an episode of Doctor Who that I really love. It's the first episode in the eleventh series. Amy Pond, the Doctor's new Companion, is living in her deceased aunt's house. She's alone, as her parents and aunt have all passed away. It's too complicated to explain here, but in her house there is a huge crack in the wall.

This is not an 'old house settling' sort of a crack. This is a monstrous crack. A portal to something evil.

Amy does not see it. I'm deliberately not using the word can't there. She is actively not looking. She instinctively knows it is something dark and dangerous, and the only way to go about her life with any sense of normalcy is to NOT SEE IT.

I am so exactly like Amy Pond. I mean, except for the being supermodel gorgeous, legs up to her chin, covet-worthy red hair, traveling through space and time with a Time Lord, thingy. Other than that we are pretty much indistinguishable.

I did it in my marriage. I was shocked when I found out the width and breadth of the deception that was going on, but somewhere - deep down - I knew something was off. I knew there was something dark lurking. I could not will myself to look at it, though. To look at it, to *know*, would require upheaval and loss. It would require change on a major level.

When I found out about the truth about my marriage my biggest wish was to not know about it. That is so humiliating to think about, much less admit publicly. I just desperately wanted to go back to not knowing, to hang onto my comfortable life.

In my attempt to stave off the pain of knowing the ugly truth, I began drinking quite a bit. I gave myself permission to drink quite a bit. I had been careful for a long time and then I stopped. I stopped being careful. After all, this terrible thing had happened. Being in the same house with my husband was excruciating, and when one is in pain one seeks anesthesia.

It became normal for me to go through a bottle of wine a night, by myself. And as the nights he came home became fewer and fewer, and I was awake, sick with worry, sometimes more.

The thing about anesthesia, though, is it numbs you to EVERYTHING. Not just pain. Joy, too.

I've always had a tricky relationship with alcohol. I drank a lot in college. I mean, a lot of people drank a lot in college, but I think I always knew I was flirting with disaster.

When I had my son and got married, it settled down. I would still have the occasional social occasion that went awry, when I would drink far too much and not remember what happened, but I wrote it off as me not going out much, not being able to handle my alcohol the way other people seemingly could.

That's true, actually. I can't. I cannot handle my alcohol the way other people can.

That is the huge, menacing, dangerous crack in the wall I had been avoiding looking at for a few years now. Somewhere along the line, I stopped drinking in response to the terrible things that were happening and just started drinking a lot. Nearly every day. My binges came closer together and not just on social occasions.

People who love me had been concerned for a while. They tried to talk to me about it, but I was not ready. I wasn't ready to look and to reach the point where I couldn't un-know. I wasn't ready for that change. I wasn't ready to never have another glass of wine. Or champagne. I admit, it makes me really sad to think about that. I loved champagne.

I just love my life more and drinking had begun to really impact my ability to live that life the way I want and to love my people the way I want. That crack that I, like Amy Pond, could only see out of the corner of my eye, was threatening to swallow me whole.

I talked to my cousin about it. I texted a friend who is in recovery. She told me not to be afraid.

I was. I was super afraid.

So I've stopped. I'm done. I am going to meetings. I walked into my first one shaking. Terrified. I was immediately approached and enveloped by some really loving women. They hugged me and held my hands, literally. They told me how things work. That I just needed to show up. That I didn't have to share until I was ready. I was not ready.

They went around the room and introduced themselves.

When it came to be my turn, I looked at the woman next to me. She smiled and nodded encouragingly. I started crying. I could barely get the words out.

"Hi, my name is Laura. I'm an alcoholic."

I cried for the rest of the meeting.

Then I went to another the next night. I've been going to meetings nearly every day since. I almost never cry anymore. In fact, I laugh at pretty much every one. Hard. And I nod my head, a lot. And I hear wisdom and I see grace. Those rooms are drenched in faith and I am soaking it up. Those rooms are Church.

I feel so much better, today. I am happier than I have ever been in my life and stronger every day. It felt like time to say it. It felt like time to tell this story. Not talking about it had begun to feel like I'm lying, and these days I do not like that feeling.

So I am going to keep going, keep learning. I am going to continue to get on my knees, every single night, and thank God for my sobriety. I'll keep doing the next right thing. I'll keep asking for help, which I still suck at - but I am getting so much better. Every day, a little better. A little more joyful. A little more healed.

And I am treating my issues like the TSA wants you to treat unattended bags. When I see something, I say something. I share my burdens, and then they are, of course, lighter.

Funny, that.

And I'll keep my eye squarely on that damned crack.

Chapter 15

Proof

"Speak softly, but carry a big can of paint."

Banksy

RECENTLY, I WAS having a conversation with a young woman who is a survivor of long-term, violent sexual abuse at the hands of a family member with whom she lived. After a series of difficult setbacks, she has found herself needing to return to live with her mother for a bit while she gets back on her feet. Her abuser is no longer alive, but she is struggling.

Every night, she's laying her head down on the very bed where she was abused as a child. She's staring at the same ceiling. She's sleeping within those same four walls.

She recounted to me the feeling she had as a young girl when she would lie in the dark and listen for footsteps. She said as bad as it was when she would hear them, the anticipation of hearing them was even worse. She said she still listens for them even though she knows they're not coming. I think about that. The terror so many of us felt in spaces that should have been our safe havens. I think about the crime scenes cleverly disguised as split-levels and subdivisions, colonials and capes, townhouses and tenements.

If a stranger rapes you in an alley, no one expects you to go back there, set up a recliner and a lamp and read the Sunday paper with your attacker. Nobody expects you to break bread with the perpetrator of a crime against you - unless it's your father, or your uncle, or your brother.

Home isn't just a structure, it's a concept. For most people, it is their soft place to fall, their safe haven. Not so, for survivors of incest. The very *IDEA* of home gets compromised. When your abuser is family, and so are his or her co conspirators or accessories after the fact, there can't be a happy homecoming. Not really. But we're expected to go home, anyway. People are asking us to pass the gravy at Thanksgiving, and we can't stop looking at the chalk outline of our childhood on the floor, the blood stains on the walls.

The crime scene tape across our bedroom doors.

She's doing it, though. She's rebuilding, leaning in, doing the work. She's a warrior.

During one of our phone conversations, she started talking about the ways her abuse played out in her life. She mentioned in an off-hand way that she was really into graffiti at one point. She said, *I don't know why I told you that, that's not really related.*

I'm not so sure about that.

I heard someone describe graffiti as aggressive once. I don't know about that, either. Aggressive is a strong word, better applied to people who ring your doorbell unexpectedly or flaunt their ability to do math. I don't think graffiti is aggressive. I think it is *insistent.*

Martin Luther King, Jr. famously said,

"Riot is the language of the unheard."

I think maybe that's true about graffiti, too. Graffiti is the *insistent* poetry of the unheard.

Multiple survivors have told me that they were very into graffiti when they were young. It makes perfect sense to me. The truth will out, but only every damned time.

I think it's another way to make your story known. We survivors are kind of brilliant, actually. At the core, these things we do as survivors, they're all the same thing. What is cutting but tagging your own body? I was here. I'm angry. I need a visible wound.

Tattoos? Storytelling murals on our very skin.

LOOK AT ME. THIS IS WHO I AM. THIS IS
HOW I FEEL.
THIS IS WHAT HAPPENED.

I have a tattoo. I got it when I was going through my divorce. I found myself sketching willow trees over and over again - something about the sinuous branches that whip and bend and snap back even when larger, seemingly stronger boughs break in the storm. Willow trees and the word *resilience*. Every pad of paper I brought with me to my lawyer's office and every awful list of assets and impossible tasks were framed in wavy branches and that word.

I talked to the tattoo artist about what I wanted and where I wanted it. I showed her what I'd sketched. I got a tattoo of the word on my spine. Not my lower back - I'm not twenty-one. The word resilience, with a willow branch running in and out of the word, along the middle of my spine. Where absolutely no one could see it. Because I, even in my attempt to tell that particular story on my skin, was keeping it secret. It's how I rolled.

The tattoo artist let me know that because of the location, because it would be directly on bone, it would likely be a little painful. Painful and permanent? That seemed right. And then she smiled and said, *I have to ask - what's the significance? There is obviously a story here.* And then, because I am super cool, I burst out crying. Full on ugly cry, shoulders heaving, nose running. Awesome.

The only words I managed to get out were, *It's just been a really hard year.*

She was so lovely to me. She sat down next to me and put her arm around me. She assured me that this happened all the time. She said that many times, people get tattoos, particularly a FIRST tattoo, at a major crossroads in their life (cue me crying harder.) She said that there are events in life that are so big, that cause such a shift in us, that we feel driven to mark the occasion. Literally. And that it is a powerful ritual.

Maybe when your wounds are invisible there's a drive to make them seen, somehow. It's like the vague disappointment you feel when you're little and you bang your knee hard on something and it hurts like hell but no bruise materializes. We want proof of harm when something hurts that much.

A few years back, I was rushing to my kid's swim meet. I was running a little late and needed to use the restroom so I ducked into the one by the gym in their high school. As I closed the door to the stall, I saw the following words written faintly in shaky handwriting on the wall. They were barely visible, but I could not tear my eyes away:

I AM NOT OK

All the hair on the back of my neck stood up. It's such a brave statement. This girl, whoever she was, was trying to find a way to tell her story.

I still find myself thinking about girl behind that graffiti all the time. It didn't strike me as someone getting a thrill out of defacing school property. That wasn't a kid trying to be a punk. I think it's the insistent handiwork of a girl who felt unseen. She could be the president of the student council, she could be the goth girl slouching through the halls, she could be the party girl who seemingly has not a care in the world. Maybe everyone thinks she's got it all together and this was her one way to let us know it's actually all falling apart. She's in the bathroom-maybe using it, maybe hiding. I hid in a lot of bathrooms in my day. And she's not okay. I hope she felt a little relief, scrawling those words on cinderblock wall.

I think about the women I work with. I think about how many of them, of us, are regularly expected to go back and visit or live or celebrate in the very houses where we were abused. I imagine if I had to go back as an adult and hang out in that utility room, the urge to make my pain known, to mark that occasion, would be pretty overwhelming. I bet a can of spray paint would feel good in my hand. I can almost feel the cool heft of it. I can envision my story writ large, paint dripping down the walls of the scene of the crime.

I WAS NOT OK.

Carrying an untold story is like trying to hold a basketball under water. You can do it for a while, but sooner or later the struggle will exhaust you and the unrelenting pressure will send it hurtling toward the surface. Keeping that story submerged indefinitely is not sustainable. It demands to be told, and if you won't tell it, it will find a way to tell itself. My story was being told by my skeletal frame, my toxic relationships, my insomnia, my striving, my control, and my drinking. All of those things were my truth making itself known; my secrets, all scrawled on the walls of the prison I'd built.

CHAPTER 16

Paper Dolls

*"There is no grater agony than bearing an
untold story inside you."*

Maya Angelou

FROM TIME TO time, I'll get an email from a reader who is not in a good place. It is almost universally a case where she tells me her life looks great from the outside, everything's shiny and happy, but she is in trouble. She is going through each day, being productive, crossing all of the things off all of the lists- being a mom, a wife, a girlfriend, a friend - a doer and a giver. She is frequently a pillar of the community: a caregiver, teacher, nurse, student, coach. She moves through her day, she smiles. She asks you, *How are YOU doing?*

Her outside, the face she shows to the world, looks great.

But if you were to really look you might see the cracks. You might notice that the bones in her wrists coming out of the oversized sweater might be just a little too pronounced. You might think, *WOW! I need to find out what diet she's on!* Or you might see her on the elliptical at the gym at a pace that seems almost manic and think, *I wish I had that commitment.*

If you came upon her in the locker room and caught her unaware, you might catch a glimpse of criss-cross scars, shiny and feathered across her belly or her thighs, maybe an angrier, more recent one. I don't know though, she's pretty careful.

If you were standing quite close to her you might pick up on the fact that her eyebrows were mostly drawn in with pencil and take note of the fact that you're pretty sure that wasn't always the case.

Our brains are miraculous. They really are. The more I talk to people, women in particular, the more I know that our pain will find a way to make itself known. As William Shakespeare put it,

"The truth will out."

I believe that when we are in such dark, low places, and the way we feel in our hearts and souls is at odds with the face we show the world, our brains try to find a way to make our outsides better match our insides.

I had this one photo as my profile picture for a while. People always comment on what a good photo it is, but that's not why I trot it out from time to time.

The day this picture was taken was one of the worst days of my life. I won't get into why - it honestly doesn't matter anymore. I was in the gorgeous backyard of my dream house, I had my two beloved dogs with me. I was wearing a cute new outfit, the sun was shining and I had a big smile on my face.

And I was dying.

I hadn't slept in I don't know how long. I was almost surely hung over. The makeup concealed dark circles under my eyes. I was wasting away. At that point, I'd probably dropped about 25 pounds in two months. The new outfit was purchased because my clothes were falling off my body. The new dog, who was an angel, was a great decision made for terrible reasons. A distraction, a band-aid on a bullet wound.

I was in serious trouble. I needed so much help.

But I was thin and I had nice clothes and a beautiful house. I had a successful husband and I was a PTA fixture. All of the messed up metrics that we use to measure well-being said I was okay. And if you'd asked me, I'd have chirped, *I'm fine! How are YOU?????* Smoke and mirrors, baby.

My veneer of 'fine-ness' was paper-thin but it looked cute and made people comfortable.

If you are not fine and are exacting some measured punishment on yourself to try and control the pain, if you are trying to disappear, or hustle, or numb, this is for you.

The rage and grief and pain need a way to come out. You've tried the other methods. You've scratched and sliced your skin to feel the manageable sting, you've felt the surge of control when you deny yourself food until you see spots, or binged in an attempt to fill the cavernous hole inside. You've bumped the acceptable hour at which to have a cocktail earlier and earlier. You've stayed up night after night until you are so tired you feel outside of your own body.

The thing is, it works for a while. The things that eventually become problems often start out as solutions. They give you the illusion that you are handling it. You're not, though, my love. You are doing the only thing your brain knows to do, at this point. You are sending out clues, whether you know it or not. Your drinking and starving and cutting and hustling are all desperate flares in the night - the problem is, not everyone understands the signals or can be bothered to decode the messages.

I know. You're thinking, *Better the pain I know. Better the pain I can control.* Maybe. But there will likely come a time when that control will become elusive. When the very things you use to manage your secrets become secrets you need to manage.

There is so much help to be had if you will just reach out for it. If you will only find someone or someplace safe to out yourself. That's no small thing, though. That's hard to do. I think we're not entwined in each other's lives enough anymore to be able to count on someone knowing when one of our tribe is fighting for their lives. Actually, too often, we don't even have tribes anymore.

A couple of years ago, I stopped hustling. I sat still for the pain. I allowed myself to feel it, I let it wash over me and I sat with it. I picked it up and turned it around in my hands. Examined it, held it close to me. Embraced it and then let it go.

It was as bad as I thought it would be. But then the unexpected happened. I lay it down, and it stayed down. It's still near me. I'm still aware of it. It's separate from me, though. It's only mine to carry now if I make the decision to pick it back up.

I wouldn't have thought that was possible. I didn't think it was possible. It is.

I read something once about this woman, a midwife. She was talking about how we do such an awful job preparing women for childbirth, particularly in this country. We either terrify them and convince they cannot possibly do what women have been doing since the beginning of time without massive intervention or we paint a rainbows and unicorns picture that does nothing to prepare them for what they are about to go through.

She takes a different approach. She says the same thing to all of her clients. *You're going to have to be brave.*

You're going to have to be a little brave, friends. If you are going to get to a place where you can lay down the dark and heavy things that are keeping you from being who you were made to be, you are going to have to be a little brave - but we already know how brave you are.

You can do this. You can stop hurting yourself. You can reach back to that little girl or boy, the one who found ways - even if they were ultimately self-destructive - to survive. You can say goodbye to the voluntary pain, to the distraction of the self-imposed wounds, and get to work on the thing. The thing you've been avoiding. The thing you've been dancing around.

The real thing. The original pain. Your darkness.

You can say, *Hello, old friend. Sit with me a while before you leave.* And it will settle on you, dark and heavy. You will feel its weight, pressing. You will fight the urge to struggle, to run, to manage it. You will sit with the pain and you will grieve the loss.

And then, acknowledged, it will lift. Bit by bit. Grudgingly, perhaps. But with patience and love and maybe a helping hand, it will go.

And then, you will rise.

Chapter 17

Messenger

"In a room where
people unanimously maintain
a conspiracy of silence,
one word of truth
sounds like a pistol shot."

Czeslaw Milosz

RECENTLY, MARY AND I were at a women's retreat telling our story and doing a workshop. We had woman after woman take us aside tell us she was doing fine, thankyouverymuch. Yes, she'd been abused, but she'd moved on. And besides, she wouldn't want to break up the family by telling the truth about what had happened to her.

It's not just at that event, either. It's the same thing over and over again. They're fine. Everybody's fine. Maybe they think about it from time to time, but it's not having any impact on their lives. It was a long time ago. Let sleeping dogs lie. It's not worth making everyone upset.

My goodness, do we make ourselves the guilty parties in our own abuse.

If it's true, that you're fine, that is *great*. What we see time and time again, though, is that once we start to talk about the ways in which our abuse affected and infected our lives people start to revisit the notion that their trauma no longer has a grip on them.

How are you sleeping? What's your relationship with food like? How is your sex life? What is your relationship with alcohol? Drugs? Do you feel the need to control everything? Are you a perfectionist? Are you in constant hustle mode - trying to be all things to all people? Are you hyper-vigilant with your kids? Are you raising them to be fearful?

When women say that to us about not wanting to break up their families by speaking the truth, we say the same thing every time, *Oh sister, your family is already broken.*

If sexual abuse is happening within your family, if the cycle of abuse and trauma is playing out on a loop from hell in your family? If your family's fate hinges on you keeping what happened to you a secret? Well, your family is fundamentally broken to begin with. It's like saying you don't want to inflict chemo on yourself because it's toxic and your body is a temple... *Honey, you have CANCER. Pick your poison.*

We hear it from women whose trauma still very much informs their lives in a myriad of ways. They have their own nuclear families, they have children of their own, but they are still pledging fealty to a family of origin that was either abusive, complicit, or so values that pretty, sparkly outside version of themselves that they are content to sacrifice one of their children at the altar of appearance, reputation, standing.

If the people in your life get angry with you for telling the truth about your abuse, that is painful and awful and great information. People really will let you know what their priorities are, one way or another.

I did a little research. The first mention of 'killing the messenger' in literature seems to be in Plutarch's Lives:

"The first messenger, that gave notice of Lucullus'
coming was so far from pleasing Tigranes that, he had
his head cut off for his pains;
and no man dared to bring further information.
Without any intelligence at all, Tigranes sat while war
was already blazing around him, giving ear only to
those who flattered him."

You know what the other title of that work is?

Parallel Lives.

Is that what you're doing? Are you living two lives? The one in the here and now, where you make no waves and pretend the smiling faces in the family portrait on the wall aren't a lie? Do you show up at your family home at the holidays, pie in hand, and pretend you aren't walking into a crime scene?

Do you spend the day frantically keeping your kids in sight, passing the potatoes, and drinking too much wine in an attempt to ignore the living, breathing dragon coiled in the corner of the room that you've all collectively agreed to pretend is pretend?

Is the other life you are leading mired in the past? You know, the past that is always present, always lurking. The flashbacks triggered by seemingly innocuous things - a snug turtleneck, a brand of soap, the smell of liquor on someone's breath.

Aren't you *tired*?

In Shakespeare's Henry IV Part II and in Antony and Cleopatra, Cleopatra threatens to tear out the messenger's eyes when told Antony has married another, eliciting the response:

> "Gracious madam, I that do bring the news made not
> the match."

No rational, healthy, non-complicit person blames a victim for telling the truth about what happened rather than the perpetrator for committing the crime to begin with. Period. And if you are still unsure, ask yourself this question: If your child was abused, if there was someone in your family or community who had preyed on your child and is likely preying on other children, would you want to know? Would you want to help and comfort your child? Would you want to protect other children? Would you want to not be in a position of welcoming your child's abuser into your home? Making them a sandwich?

None of this is your fault. Not what happened, not the aftermath. It's not your job to suffer in silence so no one has to look at the ugly, messy truth. It's not your job to smile and wave through your pain. And someone blaming you for speaking your truth is like prosecuting the person calling 911 to report a murder rather than the person who fired the gun.

I have said it before and I will keep on saying it, forever and ever amen: it is not your job to ensure that no one in your life is ever uncomfortable. It's just not. And if the cost of other people's comfort is your safety or well being?

That price is too high and it is not yours to pay.

You tell your story.

You didn't drench the house in gasoline, you didn't light the match, and you didn't toss it.

You're just calling the fire department

CHAPTER 18

Narrators

"If you are silent about your pain, they'll kill you and say you enjoyed it."

Zora Neale Hurston

I WAS TALKING to a friend last week and our conversation went deep. She was telling me some things about her past, and when she got to a certain part of her story her voice changed. It tightened. She stopped making eye contact. Her shoulders hunched. She got physically smaller.

I looked at her, this funny, smart, strong woman who I've grown to love and respect, folding in on herself. Another origami girl. I got pissed.

I held my hand up and said, *Wait. Stop.* I leaned in and asked quietly, *Who is telling your story right now?*

She looked at me, confused.

I believe babies are born loved, necessary, and enough. So that's our story when we come into the world - Loved. Necessary. Enough. The most basic of plot points.

Then our stories get entrusted to the adults in our lives. They tell our stories until we are old enough to do it ourselves.

That is an enormous amount of power to have over someone else's life, and adults have a sacred duty to wield that power with integrity and discretion.

When your story is entrusted to someone worthy of that responsibility, it's told like a great biography. These are the facts. Your praises are sung. You are reminded of your beloved-ness, your necessary-ness, your enough-ness. It's your truth. And even when there's a hard truth, even if it's something you've struggled with, failed at, need to work on, it's told with compassion and without judgment.

Those people, those trustworthy people, tell your story until you can tell it for yourself and then they hand it back to you. If you are going through a hard time, if you have forgotten who you are - that you are loved and necessary and enough - they might gently tell you your story to remind you, but they know it is not theirs to keep in the end.

The trouble is, not everyone who gets that privilege is worthy of it. Sometimes, our stories end up in the wrong hands. There's even a term for it in fiction: an unreliable narrator. That's appropriate, actually, because in the hands of an unreliable narrator our stories become works of fiction. And just because it's fiction doesn't mean it isn't hugely persuasive. Heck, I sat in the theater at the beginning of Jurassic Park and thought, *Maybe they CAN make dinosaurs out of mosquitos trapped in amber...*

Anyway, this friend and I talked some more. She asked, *How can you tell when someone else is telling your story?*

It's a great question.

In our workshops we spend time with the participants helping them to untangle the narratives of their lives, so I've been in a position to hear many women tell me their stories - and this is what I've come to believe: Anytime you feel shame - you know that hot, sick feeling in the pit of your stomach?

Anytime you feel that flush of shame, someone else is telling your story. Even if the words are coming out of your own mouth. Your story has been hijacked.

You can admit wrongdoing and not feel shame. You can have made terrible mistakes and not feel shame. Shame and guilt are very different animals. Guilt is your conscience - a giant arrow pointing to something you've done that says, *Hey! You know that was wrong. Make it right.* Guilt serves a purpose within reason. Shame does not. It is singularly destructive.

Shame is an affront to your inherent beloved-ness, it implies you are not necessary. That you can never be enough. Shame speaks in absolutes and offers no grace. Shame is always introduced by someone else. It is never indigenous.

That's actually great news, because if shame doesn't happen organically, if it is not innately part of who we are, it can be removed. Eradicated.

The first step is identifying those chapters awash in shame. The second is identifying the narrator: who is telling that part of your story? Round up the usual suspects. Then, question their stories. Stack those stories up against these three things, the bones of the story you were born with: Loved. Necessary. Enough. If the stories contradict those facts? Rewrite them.

You are the author of your life. You are. But you can only re-write a story you are willing to tell.

Until you do those things, you cannot reclaim your story. And if you don't own your story, it will own you. Guaranteed.

CHAPTER 19

Day 365

"Slowly, with many lost days, I come back to life."

Suzanne Collins

I WOKE UP this morning with a clear head and an unashamed heart. My first act, before I even opened my eyes, was to say,

"thankYouthankYouthankYouthankYouthankYouthankYouthankYou."

I say that a lot lately.

A year ago today, I walked into a church with absolutely no hope of getting sober. None. I honestly wasn't going there to get sober. I was going there because every single person in my life was upset with me. They all wanted me to try. I knew I'd been trying all day, every day, all of the days to get a handle on my drinking. Trying to control it was my full-time job. I was failing spectacularly, but it was certainly not for lack of effort. I figured at least if I went to a meeting it would finally LOOK like I was trying from the outside.

I had been trying for so long. I had no more try left in me. I was so unbelievably tired.

Laura Parrott Perry

A year ago today, I texted a friend. I said, *I'm going to my first meeting.* She replied, *What kind of meeting?* That was nice of her. I imagine her sitting, holding her phone in one hand, the fingers on the other hand crossed, whispering, *PleasedontsayWeightWatchersPleasedontsayWeightWatchers.*

I told her what kind and then said, *I'm terrified.* She texted back immediately and said, *Don't u dare be afraid. Those rooms are the only place I'm not afraid. Those are our people.*

I told her I was scared I wouldn't be able to do it.

She said, *Just promise yourself to go and sit. That's all u have to do.*

A year ago today, I decided I could probably sit in a room for an hour. Maybe.

A year ago today, I had a plan. I would walk in just minutes before the meeting started, stare down at my phone, and will no one to talk to me. My head and heart were both pounding, my hands were shaking.

A year ago today, a woman swooped down on me as soon as I walked through the door and introduced herself. She invited me to sit next to her. She was chairing the meeting, as it turns out.

So much for fading into the woodwork.

A year ago today, I hated her guts.

A year ago today, I sat around some tables while people introduced themselves.

A year ago today, I said out loud for the first time, *My name is Laura and I'm an alcoholic.* Then I burst into tears.

I remember everything about that meeting. Like my first time at hot yoga, my sole intention was to stay in the room and not throw up. I remember everyone seemed ridiculously

102

happy. When you are in despair, hope and joy are unbearable. It seemed fake. I was not buying what they were selling.

A year ago today, that same woman insisted I give her my number. A year ago today, I thought, *These people... the worst.* The next morning she set me an emoji-laden text and asked me when I was going to my next meeting. Because I was also a chronic people pleaser I didn't want to disappoint her. I consulted the Google and found another meeting so the insufferable swooper would be happy.

Today, if I had the opportunity to tweak the Beatitudes, I would add,

"Blessed are the swoopers"

A year ago tomorrow, I went to my first women's meeting and found my people. Damn it all if my friend wasn't right. I don't remember who it was and I don't remember what she said, but someone shared with such raw vulnerability and I remember having the thought - *Holy shit. We're telling the actual truth here.* It was like breathing pure oxygen after holding my breath for my entire life.

My tribe, who I now cannot imagine my life without, is full of brave, brilliant, outrageous, wildly funny, strong, tender, generous women. I see mercy, grace, and forgiveness in action every single day. It's faith with its work boots on. It is what church is supposed to be and often is not.

You know what we say when someone comes back to the rooms after they relapse? Every time? Even if it's over and over and over again? The same two things. *Welcome back. Stay.*

"Welcome back."
"Stay."

If the price of admission to this club of gloriously kind rascals is not drinking, it's a price I'll enthusiastically pay all day, every day, all the days, for the rest of my life.

I tell you what, I cannot believe I made it a year.

That's both remarkable and unremarkable simultaneously. It's remarkable in the sense that I did not for one second believe I could do it. It is unremarkable in that these 365 days do not do one single thing to guarantee me tomorrow.

I thought sobriety was something you achieve, but it isn't. That sort of sucks, but I have learned to accept it as a thing I cannot change. That's kind of a thing, as it turns out.

Sobriety is a practice, like yoga. You never have it in the bag. You never win. You never cross the finish line.

You show up every day and do the work. You tell the truth. You ask for help and you help when asked. It is as simple and hard as drinking was easy and complicated. I remember thinking in the beginning, *I cannot believe I have to do this every day.* Now I cannot believe I get to do it. I go to a meeting every day. And when everything hits the fan? When life gets super-lifey? I go to two. I look forward to them. I laugh more than I cry.

I swoop.

I've had a number of people say that sobriety seems to have come easily to me. I don't know why that is - maybe because once I stopped I stayed stopped. So far.

Hear me when I say this: I've worked for every single day of my sobriety. I fought for every minute of it and I guard it like a junkyard dog. It's far and away the hardest thing I have ever done in my life. I've learned to put my sobriety first before every other person, place, or thing in my life - because I know in my bones if I'm not sober I'll lose everything else anyway.

I wake up most mornings awash in gratitude for the opportunity to live differently and to mend what I broke. I catch glimpses of myself in mirrors or see myself in photos and there's always this little shock of recognition. I think, *There I am.* Finally

CHAPTER 20

On Harry Potter, Oprah, and Flying

*"In order to succeed, we must first believe
that we can."*

Nikos Kazantzakis

I HAVE AN app on my phone that tracks my sobriety time. Every morning it gives me my month count and a little inspirational quote. I got the one above a little while back.

I was speaking the other night and I mentioned that while I was still drinking I never, ever really thought about getting sober. Not once. Not really. Not even when everything was falling to pieces and everyone was furious with me. Not when the weight of people's disappointment was crushing, not when I knew every relationship was in jeopardy. Not even when I dragged my crushingly hungover ass to my first meeting.

I also did not spend much time contemplating learning to fly, which seemed about as likely. I knew I could not stop drinking. Knew it down to my bones. I was sure of it. How could I possibly survive life without drinking? Alcohol may have been my problem, but for a very long time, it was also my solution. Drinking was my solution to pain, to fear, to uncertainty. It worked right up until it didn't. But I honestly didn't see how I could move through the world without it. I had no reference for doing that.

I get lots of emails from readers asking about healing from abuse, so many great questions.

The other day I was asked by someone why it is that I choose to go back to the pain of my abuse over and over again, to delve back into that story. It's great that I'm in a good place with it, but having done that work why would I choose to still talk about it now? Why not put it behind me and enjoy my life rather than revisit that pain over and over again? Isn't it giving my abuser power over my life, still? And isn't it bad for me?

See? They're great questions. And I suppose questions that could also be asked about my writing about divorce and addiction.

First of all, if doing this work was bad for me I wouldn't do it. Full stop.

That's a miracle and I want everyone to take a minute to witness that. BEHOLD - A HEALTHY BOUNDARY. Isn't it beautiful? I'm thinking of having it bronzed.

This is the first time in my life when I can truthfully say that. No matter how much it might help other people, no matter how much people might want me to, no matter how much it might seem like the right thing to do, or the empowered thing to do, if revisiting my trauma on a regular basis was bad for me, I am at a place in my life where I simply would not do that.

I choose me.

I choose me and in doing so, it becomes possible for me to be of service. It's that whole putting on your own oxygen mask thing. Self care. It's a thing.

As far as giving my abuser continued control over my life, well, I just couldn't disagree more.

When I wasn't telling my story, my abuser had complete control over my life. I may not have been telling my story, but because our stories are nothing if not insistent, it was being told anyway; in addiction, eating disorders, anxiety, fearful parenting, toxic relationships, perfectionism, low self-esteem, insomnia... those things were all my story being told.

I don't know why I can revisit my trauma over and over again and not be harmed or triggered by it and I'm not sure I care much. I can. Maybe I've simply told my story so many times at this point that it's old hat. I have integrated it as *a* fact of my life, so it is no longer *the* fact of my life.

In recovery, we talk about building up a new history as a sober person. It sort of means something like this: I know I can get through this next Christmas sober because I have already done it. I've gotten through two Christmases sober. I now have that history, so, therefore, getting through Christmas without drinking is possible. That's what most people in recovery call a sober reference.

I am a massive dork, though, so instead, I always refer to Harry Potter and the Prisoner of Azkaban. Obviously.

Remember the scene when Harry, having used the Time Turner, knows he can summon his Patronus because he has already seen himself do it? (Oh, should I have said, SPOILER ALERT? Sorry. Actually - NO, I'M NOT. Read the books. See the movies. We can't all keep plots secret forever so nothing is ruined for you, precious. We're trying to live our lives here.)

Anyway, back to the Boy Who Lived. Fear couldn't lie to him and tell him it was impossible because he had proof to the contrary.

He knew he could, so he did.

Anyhow. I also believe in using other people as sober/ Harry Potter references. I know I can stay sober during terrible times because I have seen other people do so, etc. In my sober tribe I have seen people lose marriages, jobs, their health, even children, and remain sober through it, so I know it can be done.

I've had the privilege of speaking at Wild Goose a couple of times now. Do you know about the Wild Goose Festival? It's a few days in the mountains of North Carolina every summer when a bunch of beautiful hooligans get together to talk about and experience faith, justice, music, and art. Basically, all of my favorite things in life. Last summer, I had the great good fortune to hear Reverend Otis Moss III speak. That was months ago, but I'm pretty sure the trees on those mountains are still shaking.

There were two parts of his sermon that resonated deeply with me. The first was this: he spoke of our responsibility to the next person, next generation - that our sole purpose here is to open a door, create a path; make possible some opportunity for whoever is coming up behind us. Sometimes that means blazing a trail, and sometimes it just means being an example. A reference of what's possible.

After he spoke (and after I cleaned the mascara off my face) I went to his book signing. I told him what his speech had called to mind for me, in my life.

→→━● ●━←←

I have a photo from my college freshmen orientation in which I am wearing pleated dress pants, a long sleeve shirt and an enormous flowered scarf draped over one shoulder and TUCKED INTO MY PANTS in front and back, my curly hair cut short and bangs fully Aqua-Netted into submission.

Bless my heart.

I have two things to say about that.

1. It is a hand-to-God miracle that I ever made any friends at all. (Thank you, Tammy)
2. I blame Oprah.

You need only look at any Oprah episode from the 1980's to know she was the primary ~~instigator~~ inspiration for that particular fashion trend.

I could be mad about that, but it seems ungrateful given that Oprah Winfrey saved my life.

I am well aware I am not the only person to say such a thing, but it's a fact.

True story.

It was spring of my freshman year and I was perched on the corner of my next-door neighbor's narrow dorm bed on the seventh floor of International Hall. We were watching Oprah because it was 1989 and that's what you did.

I can't remember exactly what the episode was about, but I remember at one point she began speaking about her sexual abuse. I got very still. Typically, in the exceedingly rare event the subject of sexual abuse was raised, my go-to response was to flee. This time was different.

The reason I froze, the reason I didn't hastily excuse myself, was the way Oprah talked about it. She didn't avert her eyes. She didn't lower her voice, or apologize for talking about her experience. She just said it. She was factual.

She was shameless.

Now, it's not like I had some magical moment and my shame just fell away. I had to do the work. And it's not like I had the thought, *Ohmigosh - Oprah and I are so exactly alike, therefore, I can be shameless, too!* I mean, she's OPRAH, for heaven's sake. But up until that moment, perched on the corner of that dorm bed avoiding eye contact with the other girls in the room, it had quite simply never occurred to me that shamelessness was an option. Oprah telling her story without shame allowed for that possibility. She created that space in my world - a space I was nowhere near ready to inhabit, mind you - but now it existed.

Those sober, Harry Potter/Oprah references are at least as important as the cautionary tales everyone always wants you to heed. The ones that tell you why it won't work, why you can't, what could happen. I even hear survivors utter these words of warning or fear about the process of healing, as though leaning into that pain is too daunting. That they can't delve into the pain of their past, it's too much. Too painful. Too treacherous.

That's a big part of why I do what I do - because we need models of life after trauma. We need to know that shamelessness, health, healing, and joy are possible. We need to SEE it, because it seems impossible. When you are stuck in it, you might as well obsess about learning to fly.

It can get so much better, though. It can. This I can promise you, the work to heal will not be worse than the wound, and you already survived that.

CHAPTER 21

Lovely Little Deaths

"Why do you stay in prison
when the door is so wide open?"

Rumi

AUTUMN HAS ALWAYS been my favorite season. I live in New England, and autumn in New England is spectacular. The impossibly crisp, blue-skied days, the smell of woodsmoke at night, and the brilliantly colored foliage that draws people from all over the country to drive 25 mph in a 55 mph zone. #JesusFixIt

I love the fall. I am energized by it. I tend to start new projects, set new goals. It's a very productive time for me, creatively, and yet there's also a fairly deep vein of melancholy for me at this time of year.

Wistfulness has always been a part of my make-up, even though I'm generally a positive person. I always wondered why that was. Why, during a season that delights me so much, do I experience waves of something akin to grief?

I recently read something in a book about different seasons serving different purposes in our lives. It posited that the fall is a good time to take stock of where you are at, what you need to work on, what you have, and what you no longer need. An inventory, if you will. Now that may seem like a task more suited to spring, but the more I thought about it, the more it made sense. I also read a few articles about the Eastern perspective on seasons. They said that in Chinese philosophy the emotions most closely associated with autumn are courage and sadness.

That feels right to me.

All seasons are transitions when you think about it. If winter is a season of dormancy and gestation, and springtime is a season of newness and birth, then really, autumn, at its heart, is a season about dying.

All those beautiful leaves that the out of town peepers come to ogle?

Thousands upon thousands of lovely, necessary little deaths.

This brings us to the second part of Reverend Moss' Wild Goose sermon that has stayed with me. He was talking about the constant hand-wringing over the belief that the American church is dying. His take on it?

Then LET. IT. DIE. Some things need to die.

He went on to talk about how things need to die in order for something else to be birthed - something new, something better. Something closer to who we are intended to be.

I've been thinking about this a lot in terms of trauma and what we do with it. I think in order to truly heal we must be willing to let some things die.

Human beings are story-making creatures. As long as humans have existed, so has story. Since the beginning of time, we've sought to make sense of the world by taking the some-times mystifying facts at hand and building story around them. The volcano erupted? The gods are angry. A bountiful harvest? Our sacrifices pleased the gods. An independent woman? Must be a witch.

When we endure trauma as children, we have neither the life experience nor the wisdom to put it into any kind of healthy context. We don't know enough about the world or human na-ture or the way people and institutions are supposed to behave to frame our abuse appropriately. And frequently, our abusers are people we trust, even love; people who we believe to be infallible or all-powerful. That emotional and spiritual disso-nance lends itself perfectly to story-building.

Children take a complicated situation and make a simple story out of it. As little kids, we take the facts of our abuse, use them as scaffolding and then we build walls of story around them. We build a house out of that story and we live in it.

And even when the stories we build are overwhelmingly harmful, we can be reluctant to let them go.

I think we sometimes cling to long-held beliefs about our trauma and what it means because to challenge the validity of those beliefs is to set our houses on fire. It's a death. And even if the story you've been living out of is dark and toxic and pain-ful? It might be a prison but it's also home.

In his brilliant book, Finding God in the Ruins: How God Redeems Pain, Matt Bays reminds us that redemption is, by definition, an exchange. In order to write a new ending for your story, you may need the willingness to offer up long-held assumptions, beliefs, and identities at the altar of healing. Maybe you have to turn in your notion of what your life is supposed to look like in order to be sober. Maybe you need to trade in your long-held internalization of society's idea of a woman's beauty and worth in order to have a healthy relationship with your body. Maybe what you exchange in return for freedom from your trauma is the story you've lived in since you were abused.

What are you waiting for? Do you think tomorrow is guaranteed? How much time have you sacrificed in order to guard the house of pain you live in? Has it maybe been long enough? Look around at your story-house. Has it become a prison? If it has, and the walls are the secrets you're keeping and the story you told yourself about what your abuse meant about you, your family, the world, God... here's the good news: Those walls may be tall and seemingly impenetrable, but the door is WIDE OPEN. You need only decide to walk out.

If your old story needs to die for you to heal, then *let it die*.

Maybe this is the season for that. Drag it out into the sunlight and let it die, like the scarlet and gold drifts against the fence outside my window. Let the story in which you've been serving time die a lovely little death. It's necessary.

Toss a match and let it burn, like so many brilliantly colored leaves. Stand in the waning autumn light and breathe in the smoke. Hold courage in one hand and sadness in the other. Only then can you write a new ending. You really can, you know. You can strip away all that story, go back to the bones, the facts, and build yourself a new home.

Conclusion

"The small woman
Builds cages for everyone
She
Knows.
While the sage,
Who has to duck her head
When the moon is low,
Keeps dropping keys all night long
For the
Beautiful
Rowdy
Prisoners"

Hafiz

HUMAN BEINGS HAVE lived inside stories since before we lived inside houses. We're not just storytellers - it's deeper than that. We're story-dwellers. Story is what we use to make sense of the sometimes-mystifying world. Story is how we bring order to things.

We also build our lives out of story and when we decide those stories are unspeakable, we build prisons out of our secrets. The stories we get told and sold in childhood become the foundation of our lives, for better or for worse.

The stories we create to make sense of things become real for us. We live inside them. Your house is not your home – your story is. We think we build walls to protect ourselves, but eventually they imprison us. When our stories are secrets we stack them high until we're trapped behind them. You know what the difference between a home and a prison is? It's just your ability to step outside it to freedom.

A story untold is static. It cannot be changed, it cannot be altered. It's what T.S. Eliot called a still point. Neither past nor present. Secrets are about the past, but they cannot remain there because we doggedly carry them with us.

My history was just that - literally, HIS STORY. History is generally the record of what happened as written by the victors. For the longest time, my history was written by my abuser. I ceded victory to him and allowed him to frame the narrative of my life. Because I would not do my work and rid myself of my secrets, I ceased to be the protagonist in my own life story. Life was happening to me. I was a victim, an adjunct character, a bit player.

I think more often than not, people don't just create stories - stories create people.

In order to reclaim our stories, in order for them to be redeemed, they must be told.

You can lay your secrets down. You don't need to carry them around forever. Once acknowledged and processed, our shame stories lose their grip on us. Shame can only exist in the dark. Once you tell your story, you begin to reclaim it.

I've learned many things in the past few years, nothing more important than this: Whatever pain or fear I don't share, I feed. Whatever story I try to hide becomes more powerful.

The second, and I mean the second I feel that feeling - that hot, sick tug of shame in my stomach, I know I need to say it out loud. I need to give voice to it. I need to name the narrator.

And I know this is easier said than done. I know the fear of being seen and of people knowing you for you - who you really are - can be terrifying. Truly. I know that paralyzing fear. I know the very real apprehension of not wanting to ring a bell that can never be un-rung. I know what it's like to worry, *If I share this part of my story, that's all the other person will ever see when they look at me, they'll never see me the same way again.* I know how it feels to fear, *If I say this thing out loud I might shatter into a million pieces.*

You know what? You might. You might shatter into a million pieces - but trust me on this: broken and irreparable are not synonyms. I know the fear and anxiety and shame and feeling of being exposed seem like they could kill you, but they can't. You know what can? Shame. Shame can kill you. Shame has a body count attached to it. There's a reason we use the word survivor, you know. It's because not all of us do. Not all of us survive. And the ones that don't are almost always the ones who never found a way to tell their story.

I work with people every day who have done everything possible to keep their secrets. They sign up for every voluntary pain in order to not feel *the* pain. They drink, they drug, they eat, they starve, they strive, they shop, they gamble, they use sex, they cut - and it's all the same damned thing - they're trying anything and everything to avoid telling their story and feeling the pain of it. I want to say to them,

> "Honey, you survived the THING,
> you sure as HELL can survive TALKING about the thing."

If you're not okay, find a way to say it, like that girl in the bathroom stall. I had someone really wise say to me once, *If there's a word for what you did or what happened to you, that means you didn't invent it.* Whatever the thing is, I promise you are not alone in it.

You don't have to tell your story publicly. You don't have to write a book or go on TV. You don't have to stand on a stage. My way doesn't need to be your way.

Hear me when I say this: Your story matters. It does. And if it is going untold because you've decided it's unspeakable, then I have news for you - you aren't keeping secrets - your secrets are keeping you. Keeping you stuck. Sick. Lonely. Afraid. *What will the world miss if you don't tell your story?*

It'll miss YOU.

You do not owe anyone the tidy, edited version of yourself. You were not put here to be small and convenient, to round the edges of your truth so no one's neatly stitched comfort gets snagged on it and unravels.

You are not what happened to you. That darkness is not yours to carry alone. Your truth is only a life sentence if you impose it on yourself. Our untold stories, our untreated traumas? They get weaponized. We turn them inward or we turn them outward, but a knife is a knife is a knife, whether we cut ourselves or someone else.

Drop your weapons. Tell your story.

⋅⇥⇥◉ ◉⇤⇤⋅

I look out into the audience. My eyes are clear. Focused.

I take a deep, easy breath and then I introduce myself.

I am no longer wracked by fear of speaking to crowds and I am no longer afraid to be seen. Invariably, I find that when I am standing on that stage or in that tent, or sitting in that circle, the parts of my story that I'd attached the most shame to, the parts of my story I thought were the unspeakable chapters - too awful to give voice to - are the parts that shift the energy in the room.

I am a survivor of sexual abuse.
I couldn't stop drinking.
I was a terrible mother.
I never thought I was enough.
I was starving myself.
I did so much harm.
I didn't say no.
My heart was broken.
I felt forsaken.
I was so lonely.
I was so afraid.
I wanted to die.

That's when I see heads nod. That's when I see eyes well up in recognition. That's when I see, *me too.* That's when connection happens - in those moments.

And I see it. I see it because I am no longer glazing my eyes over to avoid that connection. I'm seeking it. I'm looking for the eyes that are seeking mine and I am looking for the eyes that are averted.

I see you, I think to myself.

I can see you because I am willing to be seen. I can hear your stories because I am willing to tell mine.

⟶▬◉ ◉▬⟵

Sometimes when I post on my blog, I'll see a bunch of sad emojis in the Facebook notifications. I always have a moment of, *Oh no! What are people sad about?* There's always a moment of surprise when I realize it's in response to part of my story.

I don't think of my story that way. I'm not sad. Not today. Not even when I am delving back into those stories of pain. I live joyfully today, even when things are hard. It would be a disservice to that little girl who fought and struggled and suffered not to do so. That perspective didn't just happen, of course. There's no magic wand. Just work. Just telling my stories and doing the work around them. And while that work is difficult, it doesn't seem like a lot to ask for on behalf of that scrappy eight-year-old who somehow found a way to survive.

I had an editor – a really lovely, kind, smart person – advise me against writing this particular book. I was cautioned against having my first book be "a lament." I know what he meant. He was trying to be helpful. A person can be both deeply good and really wrong about something, just the same way someone can be bad and right.

The good news is this; I no longer rely on other people to tell me what my story is. In telling my story, I now understand it more fully. This story is absolutely not a lament. My story is a story that has some hard chapters, but ultimately, it is a story of healing and grace and redemption.

I should know. I am writing it.

> But my story is only now beginning
> Don't try to write my ending
> Nobody gets to sing my song...

⤚▬◉ ◉▬⤙

> And this hill is not the one I die on
> I'm going to lift my eyes and
> I'm going to keep on climbing
> This is the sound of surviving
> This is my farewell to fear
> This is my whole heart deciding
> I'm still here, I'm still here

Nichole Nordeman

Acknowledgements

To my kids. You are far and away the best gifts I have to offer. It's not even close. I love you, I love you, I love you, I love you. This world is so much better because you're in it. I hit the jackpot with you two, hand to God.

To Stephen. You really are my Favorite. Thank you for never wanting me to be small or quiet and for always, always having my back. I love us.

To Thing One and Littlest. I'm so blessed to be a part of your lives. You are the best bonuses. Love you.

To Angela, the Gravy to my Mashed Potatoes. You are so good at loving your people. I thank God every day I am one of them.

To Mary. Thank you for everything. All of the things. I'm profoundly grateful to have you back in my life. Your support and love is unparalleled. I'd walk into a police station with you any day, sister. I'll call you in five minutes.

To MattBaysLifeCoach. Our friendship is proof positive that God loves me and wants the best for me. I am filled with gratitude to have had your input while writing this. You knock me out, brother. Please always tell me the truth about my eyebrows.

To Jessica Faith Kantrowitz. Thank you for your enormously helpful feedback and steadfast love, and for quite simply being one of the very best people I know. The coffee pot is full, sister. Always.

To Officer Paul Smith. Thank you for writing it down and for being a constant reminder of how much good can come of the simple act of bearing witness. Say It, Survivor exists because you heard our story with respect and treated us with dignity. We'll just keep thanking you forever and ever, okay?

To Rachel Macy Stafford for her relentless encouragement and for always reminding me to lead with love.

To Glennon Doyle and Jen Hatmaker for helping introduce He Wrote it Down to the world so eventually She Wrote it Down could find her own way.

To my Room sisters - my writing hive mind. So grateful for your guidance, advice, encouragement, and laughter.

To my Wednesday Women and my Morning Crew. Thank you for saving my life every day. And to LB, for helping to make it a life worth saving.

To my Say It, Survivor community. It is the great honor of my life to bear witness to your stories and to serve you. I hold you in my heart every day.

To my mother. Thank you for believing me and believing in me.

To my sisters - my first friends, my life-long confidantes, my eternal co-conspirators. You are the constant.

To the guiding lights and writers, including those named above, whose work inspires and challenges me, and whose writing can be found within the pages of this book and on my blog. I am, as ever, inspired by what I find in others' words. Some of you helped me write, some of you helped me get sober, and some of you are just North Stars. Maya Angelou, Oprah Winfrey, Anne Lamott, Brené Brown, Nadia Bolz-Weber, J.K. Rowling, Shauna Niequist, Rob Bell, Mary J. Blige, Alanis Morissette, Jonathan Martin, Elizabeth Gilbert, Shawn Colvin, Toni Morrison, Rachel Held Evans, Alice Walker, Zora Neale-Hurston, John Green, Cheryl Strayed, Donald Miller, and a million I'm forgetting, but who have, nonetheless, shaped me as a woman and a writer. I learned to tell stories by reading those written by the likes of them.

About the Author

Laura Parrott Perry is the author of the popular eponymously named blog (formerly known as In Others' Words) and The Golden Repair on DivorcedMoms.com. Her work has been featured on The Huffington Post, in Boston Magazine, on Trigger Points Anthology, and No Make-Up Required. Laura is a frequent public speaker on the topics of shame, trauma, addiction, and story. She has been a contributor at The Wild Goose Festival and a guest on numerous podcasts, including Poema, Spiritual Charlotte, The Practical Minimalists and A Wish Come Clear's 'You Need to Read' series. She is co-founder and CEO of Say It, Survivor; a non-profit committed to helping survivors of child sexual abuse reclaim their stories.

Laura is the mother of two phenomenal human beings, a former art teacher, painter, and devoted servant to a Perfect dog. She also has another dog. He is Bad. She lives by the beach in Connecticut with her family.